Occupational Health & Safety, Some Recent Court Decisions

By

Patricia E.A. Mallenby, BA, BSc

And

Jeremy T.T. Mallenby, BA, BSc

References courtesy of the Fair Use Act, for research purposes, to clarify the author's point of view.

The 1961 Report of the Register of Copyrights on the General Revision of the U.S. Copyright Law cites examples of activities that courts have regarded as fair use:

> *"quotation of excerpts in a review or criticism for purposes of illustration or comment; quotation of short passages in a scholarly or technical work, for illustration or clarification of the author's observations; use in a parody of some of the content of the work parodied; reproduction of a work in legislative or judicial proceedings ..."*

Preface

There are some terrific courses out-there in the field of Occupational Health & Safety, and some of the precautions one needs to take at work, in the environment and in your personal life.

One example is:

Steven Geigle, M.A., CIT, CET, CSHM
OSHAcademy Occupational Safety and Health Training
515 NW Saltzman Road #767
Portland, Oregon 97229-6098
http://webcache.googleusercontent.com/search?q=cache:Lg-
kbz_occYJ:www.oshatrain.org/+degree+programs+occupational+health+%26+safety&
cd=3&hl=en&ct=clnk&gl=ca&source=www.google.ca

This little book is about some of them.

It also emphasizes the need, in such a world we find ourselves, it pays for everyone to take personal precautions for themselves, their families, and their loved ones.

Jeremy T.T. Mallenby, BA, BSc

and

Patricia E.A. Mallenby, BA, BSc

Index

Chapter 1 – That old boy's club mentality

In the course 700 Intro to Safety Management[1], it is empasized "management commitment to safety will occur to the extent each manager clearly understands the positive benefits derived from their effort. Understanding the benefits will create a strong desire to improve the company's safety culture."[2]

Unfortunately, not all employers value all of their employees.

Take for example the hazardous working environments some female police officers have had to put up with? As cited in "Perverts, Sexual Deviants Occupy Top RCMP Ranks"[3], "allegations Say Some Top Officers Constantly Harassed Women Officers For Sex, Blackmailed Some Trainees Into Sexual Submission – Their Punishment A Slap On The Wrist If Caught!"[4]

In other situations, such wanton behavior has put the general public in danger. These "serious allegations of sexual harassment, blackmailing trainees into sexual submission and corruption have come to light against top RCMP officers, some of whom were involved in the expensive Air India investigation, which was dodged by failure on the part of the force, as well as another troubling investigation of sex-killer Robert Willy Pickton."[5]

In fact, "more female members of the RCMP in British Columbia have come forward with serious allegations of harassment following CBC News's shocking revelations of well-known Mountie spokeswoman Cpl. Catherine Galliford 's claims she suffered from years of sexual harassment."[6]

As cited by Brown & Fielding (1993), "there are relatively few differences in exposure to organizational stressors except that women detectives and uniformed officers report higher rates of sex discrimination and prejudice than policemen."[7]

Similarly, Wexler & Logan (1983) found that female police officers "frequently commented that 'the department doesn't want women.' The subjects generally perceived that after 6 years on patrol, they were still not accepted as officers. They considered themselves to be ignored, harassed, watched, gossiped about, and viewed as sexual objects."[8]

Paula Brough & Rachael Frame (2004) emphasized the importance of supervisor support, "the retention of operational staff, particularly females, within the police services and other male-dominated occupations, has received some recent attention ... The importance of adequate supervisor support is one such intervention and has produced considerable recent interest."[9]

Quite clearly, apparently none of these female Royal Canadian Mounted Police officers received any such support; as reported, Female RCMP officer "Galliford said she experienced six to 10 incidents of harassment or sexual harassment, including one occasion in which a superior showed her his genitals and asked if a mole on his penis was 'cute'."[10]

"Following Galliford's explosive allegations, Krista Carle contacted CBC News, breaking her own long silence."[11]

"I know for a fact there are at least six women that I know [who] have left the force or are still in that have suffered harassment," Carle said. "I'm sure there are others who are afraid to come forward for fear of reprisals."[12]

"Carle, who graduated from the RCMP's training academy with Galliford in 1991, says she was harassed and sexually assaulted. She is now off the job and says she has been diagnosed with post-traumatic stress disorder." [13]

"RCMP management tried to cover up the problems when she complained, Carle told CBC News."[14]

"When I spoke out against the harassment, it wasn't taken seriously and I felt diminished and I felt re-victimized every time I told what happened to me," she said.[15]

In other situations, the first female security officer hired for the forensic psychiatric unit of Selkirk Mental Health Centre in Manitoba, Canada was subject to discrimination with virtually no support from her supervisor. [16]

For example, as cited in her Manitoba Human Rights Commission complaint: [17]

-12 December 2010, S.F. knowing full well that SMHC has a 'same sex' search policy still protested to my supervisor [B.L.] that I was not searching male patients / visitors, and even held everyone up because he had to email [B.L.] right away to make a [bogus] complaint, while the PNAs were 'demanding' he hurry up with his email to [B.L.] [incident cited in my evidence book, and mentioned in email to CEO dated 09 January 2011].

-Around the same time, B.S. said to me that "if I couldn't do male searches than why bother (doing the job)" [mentioned in email to CEO dated 09 January 2011].

-On 24 December 2010 when C.D. told me to stay out of the control room, go on patrol so to keep busy I spent a good number of hours doing patrols; I was on patrol from 11:50 to 16:45 in the frigid cold [incident cited in my evidence book, and mentioned in email to CEO dated 09 January 2011].

[Note: a control room roster was implemented by the CEO to prevent anyone, including C.D. from hogging the control room].

-On 29 December 2010 C.D. again told me to stay out of the control room so to keep busy I again spent a good number of hours doing foot patrols, from 09:00 to 14:25 in the frigid cold [incident cited in my evidence book, and mentioned in email to CEO dated 09 January 2011].

-29 December 2010 my supervisor [B.L.] mentioned that he had [bogus] complaints from C.D. that I was not searching male patients / visitors, some of the complaints apparently dating back to October 2010 and these could lead to my dismissal [see my emails dated 30 December 2010, 31 December 2010, 02 January 2011, 03 January 2011all sent to my supervisor B.L. with no answer from B.L. about these bogus complaints].

- 08 January 2011, J.Mat. when he found out I was coming in for a 'sick' shift said: "Why is she coming in"; "She can't do anything"; "I have to do the searches" (i.e., the male searches); "We don't want any female SO ... as they cannot do the work" (i.e., search male patients / visitors) [incident cited in another S.O.'s evidence book, and mentioned in email to CEO dated 09 January 2011].

[Note: a call-in roster was implemented by the CEO to ensure everyone got an equal crack at available shifts, although people like J.Mat. still seem to be circumventing it]

-08 January 2011 when I arrived on duty I was told by J.Mat. to stay out of the control room because he was busy playing with his 'ipod' and 'lap top' [mentioned in email to CEO dated 09 January 2011].

Yes, I would like to proceed to investigation. With what I have accumulated, the witnesses I have at my disposal [in letter form], and documents and materials MHRC can glean during their investigation should do the trick to confirm sex discrimination / unequal treatment against me as the first casual female Security Officer hired at SMHC.[18]

Even the Female RCMP received no support; as further noted, "Sexual harassment of women thrives in environments that are male dominated, hierarchal and demand strict adherence to codes of silence like the RCMP," said MacDougall, noting female officers are afraid to speak up.[19]

In a 115-page statement to RCMP Internal Affairs Insp. Paul Darbyshire, Galliford said she documented the sexual harassment she experienced from top RCMP."[20]

An RCMP boss insisted she go along on road trips to visit victims' families "and then he'd turn into Octopus-Man in a hotel room at night," she said.[21]

Galliford named another female officer who had to physically fight off "an attempted rape" by the same officer. Female civilians also were targeted.[22]

Galliford is also haunted by the fact that senior officers appeared to know that now-convicted serial killer Robert Pickton was a "prime suspect" in the murder of Downtown Eastside sex workers at his Port Coquitlam pig farm.[23]

One of the problems with research in this field is highlighted by Albert (1984) where he states: "social scientists have a unique opportunity to generate empirical data to assist legal arguments in a court of law. Unfortunately, most researchers seldom take the initiative to research specific issues that may guide a legal question. Instead, they research issues that may interest them but have no real-world application."[24]

However, Simpson, McCarrey & Henry (1987) apparently pin-pointed an old-boys club mentality or the "traditional" supervisors of staff: "traditional supervisors of women … compared to traditional supervisors of men, evaluated the women supervised, even in the face of substantial direct contact, as less able to: (1) autonomously direct their subordinates; (2) assist in the career development of their subordinates; and (3) effectively monitor the day-to-day results of their subordinates."[25]

Continuing, "compared to egalitarian supervisors, traditional supervisors were reluctant to assign technical, vital high-profile projects to female subordinates. The results were interpreted in terms of mores from the greater macro-culture which were reflected inside the organization via gender-related barriers to equity such as absence of effective role models, difficulty gaining access to informal networks, tokenism, and the belief found here that women as supervisors in non-traditional areas are dysfunctional for the organization and for the upward mobility of their subordinates."[26]

A multitude of articles and books have been written about this "old boy's club" mentality!

For example, Zhuge et. al. (2011) found, "despite the dramatically increased entry of women into general surgery and surgical subspecialties, traditionally male-dominated fields, there remains a gross under-representation of women in the leadership positions of these departments."[27]

Unfortunately, very few organizations do anything about it – such as, apparently, the Royal Canadian Mounted Police? As cited, "as a retired member of the RCMP, I have nothing but respect for Catherine Galliford coming forward and exposing the truth about harassment in the force."[28]

"The RCMP may have very strict harassment policies in place, and on paper they may look good, but that does not change the fact that it is an old boy's club and once word of a an allegation gets out, and it will, it will follow you for the rest of your career and only lead to more harassment."[29]

"I speak from experience and I applaud Galliford's bravery, as should all women on the force and any other women and men who experience workplace harassment."[30]

It appears that neither the Manitoba Government or the Government of Canada have noted the statistics on workplace bullying, and have done nothing about it:

"Poll Suggests that Bullying is Pervasive at Work"
July 14, 2010
Michael Fitzgibbon
http://labourlawblog.typepad.com/managementupdates/2010/07/poll-suggests-that-bullying-is-pervasive-at-work.html

In light of the coming into force of Ontario's Bill 168, violence and harassment in the workplace is (or should be) front of mind for employers in this province. It should be front of mind for employers even without legislation.

As reported in HR Magazine Bullying remains rife in the workplace. According to the article a recent poll suggests that "more than one in five of respondents (21%) feel 'bullied' by their boss at work and a further 28% feel picked on by a co-worker in the office"

As further reported:

One in three people bullied at work
Tom Newcombe , 16 Nov 2012
http://www.hrmagazine.co.uk/hro/news/1075371/one-people-bullied

One in three people have suffered some form of bullying at work, according to a survey by One Poll. The survey revealed that 43% of those bullied do nothing about it and 1 in 10 of them are forced to leave their job due to bullying.

Dr Catherine Sandler, director at executive coaching firm, Sandler Consulting said: "Bullying is a destructive feature of working life that has proved extremely difficult to eradicate since it was first highlighted in the early 1990s. "When challenged, the bully is usually defensive, denying their behaviour or placing the responsibility on others. They reject the accusation of bullying and often feel furious that the organisation to which they give so much is attacking them." Sandler added: "HR has a vital role to play in this process. Those organisations who find the courage and skill to put a stop to bullying reap a huge return on their investment. Not only will the morale and performance of staff be transformed but the former bully will also raise their contribution to a new level."

Jan Parkinson, chief executive of the Employee Relations Institute (ERI), said: "Bullying is just one issue that results from poor employee engagement, ultimately effective and meaningful employee engagement is crucial in improving workplace relations." Parkinson added: "Organisations with engaged employees not only experience less bullying, but also find there is higher productivity and better staff retention. The key is better training and awareness at all levels of the organisation." With 40% of those surveyed feeling unsupported by their line manager, the survey claims it is clear that the importance of effective management capability and employee engagement must be highlighted and improved. Andy Cook, executive chair at ERI, told HR magazine: "I'm not surprised by the findings but I don't believe the figure of 1 in 3 is all serious bullying.

"If a manager has to deal with a bullying complaint they must investigate with the utmost urgency and the investigation has to be thorough. If they don't look at every aspect they could be accused of covering something up."

Footnotes

1 - 2. *700 Intro to Safety Management*
Steven J. Geigle, MA, CET, CSHM
OSHAcademy Safety and Health Training
www.oshatrain.org

3 – 6. *Perverts, Sexual Deviants Occupy Top RCMP Ranks – New Allegations Suggest*
Saturday, November 12th, 2011
http://thelinkpaper.ca/?p=11604

Also see: *Female RCMP officers' accounts of sexual harassment in force prompt new hotline*
By Suzanne Fournier, The Province November 25, 2011
http://www.theprovince.com/news/Female+RCMP+officers+accounts+sexual+harassment+force+prompt+hotline/5763916/story.html

7. Jennifer Brown & Jane Fielding, "Qualitative differences in men and women police officers' experience of occupational stress", *Work & Stress*, Volume 7, Issue 4, 1993.

8. J.G. Wexler & D.D. Logan, "Sources of Stress Among Women Police Officers", *Journal of Police Science and Administration*, Volume 11(1), March 1983, pp. 46-53.

9. Paula Brough & Rachael Frame, "Predicting Police Job Satisfaction and Turnover Intentions: The Role of Social Support and Police Organisational Variables", *New Zealand Journal of Psychology*, Vol. 33, 2004

Also see: Kate Sparks, Brian Faragher & Cary L. Cooper, "Well-being and occupational health in the 21st century workplace", *Journal of Occupational and Organizational Psychology*, Volume 74, Issue 4, pages 489–509, November 2001.

10 - 15. *Perverts, Sexual Deviants Occupy Top RCMP Ranks – New Allegations Suggest* Saturday, November 12th, 2011
http://thelinkpaper.ca/?p=11604

Also see: *Eighty-one cases of misconduct by Mounties*. By The Vancouver Sun October 15, 2006.
http://www.canada.com/vancouversun/news/story.html?id=f6b8fe2d-e802-4817-aefe-d0b47a086dc2&k=58373

Also see: *RCMP scandals and setbacks since 2006*. Globe and Mail Update. Published on Thursday, Mar. 29, 2007, Last updated on Tuesday, Mar. 31, 2009.
http://www.theglobeandmail.com/news/national/article750473.ece

16 - 18. *Black Balled by Manitoba Government for making sex-discrimination complaint* http://www.amazon.com/BLACK-BALLED-Manitoba-Government-sex-discrimination/dp/1466480890/ref=sr_1_32?s=books&ie=UTF8&qid=1320313966&sr=1-32

Also see: *Walking amongst the cannibals! Watching out for the sharks?* http://www.amazon.com/Walking-amongst-cannibals-Watching-sharks/dp/146647291X/ref=sr_1_30?s=books&ie=UTF8&qid=1320314090&sr=1-30

19 23. *Female RCMP officers' accounts of sexual harassment in force prompt new hotline*
By Suzanne Fournier, The Province November 25, 2011
http://www.theprovince.com/news/Female+RCMP+officers+accounts+sexual+harassment+force+prompt+hotline/5763916/story.html

24. Geoffrey P. Alpert, "The Needs of the Judiciary and Misapplications of Social Research The Case of Female Guards in Men's Prisons", *Criminology*, Volume 22, Issue 3, pages 441–456, August 1984.

25 - 26. Suzanne Simpson, Michael McCarrey & P. Henry, "Relationship of Supervisors' Sex-Role Stereotypes to Performance Evaluation of Male and Female Subordinates in Non-traditional Jobs", *Canadian Journal of Administrative Sciences / Revue Canadienne des Sciences de l'Administration*, Volume 4(1), pp. 15 – 30, March 1987.

27. Zhuge, Ying; Kaufman, Joyce; Simeone, Diane; Chen, Herbert; Velazquez, Omaida, "Is There Still a Glass Ceiling for Women in Academic Surgery?" *Annals of Surgery*, April 2011, Volume 253(4), pp. 637 – 643.

Also see: Backhouse, Constance "Chilly Climate for Women Judges: Reflections on the Backlash from the Ewanchuk Case", *Canadian Journal of Women and the Law*, Volume 15(1), Number 1, 2003, p.167

Also see: Santoro, Rachel "Narrowing the Cat's Paw: An Argument for a Uniform Subordinate Bias Liability Standard", U. Pennsylvania Journal of Business Law, Volume 11(3), 2008-2009.

Also see: Margaret Alston, *Breaking Through Grass Ceiling: Women, Power and Leadership in Agricultural Organisations*. Routledge: Studies in Management, Organizations and Society, 2000.

28 - 30. "Province Letters: RCMP sexual harassment, Occupy Vancouver, Carol Berner, Mayor Dianne Watts, Christy Clark", November 11, 2011
http://blogs.theprovince.com/2011/11/11/province-letters-rcmp-sexual-harassment-occupy-vancouver-carol-berner-mayor-dianne-watts-christy-clark/

Chapter 2 – No reply from supervisor

In the course 700 Intro to Safety Management[1], it is further emphasized "a safety policy may be mandatory (a rule) or voluntary (a guideline). It is a predetermined (usually written) statement that provides direction in decision making. It reflects top management goals and objectives related to the safety function within the company. An effective safety policy is both educational and directive. It informs everyone about expected safety behaviors and standards and why they are important. It also assigns responsibility to perform certain duties or oversee people and programs."[2]

It's very clear that inadequate organizations are lacking in this category. Just as the first female security officer hired at Selkirk Mental Health Centre did not hear from her immediate supervisor [B.L.][3] neither did the female RCMP officers when they complained to higher-ups?[4]

As reported previously, "RCMP management tried to cover up the problems when she complained, Carle told CBC News."[5]

"When I spoke out against the harassment, it wasn't taken seriously and I felt diminished and I felt re-victimized every time I told what happened to me," she said.[6]

It's very apparent, the Manitoba Government in Canada has not learned sufficiently about bullying at work, or has not bothered to correct the behavior:

Tackling the explosive bully
Catherine Sandler , 12 Dec 2012
http://www.hrmagazine.co.uk/hro/features/1075697/tackling-explosive-bully

Bullying is a destructive feature of working life that has proved extremely difficult to eradicate since it was first highlighted in the early 1990s. Bullying can cause immense harm. Apart from the human cost, employers risk litigation, expensive settlements and reputational damage. This article explores the emotional dynamics behind one of the most widespread forms of bullying and how HR can help address this critical issue. The psychopathic bully Before tackling a bully, it is important to recognise that a small but significant number have personalities which fall on the psychopathic or personality-disordered spectrum. Focused solely on their own interests, they lack integrity, an internal moral compass or the capacity to empathise.

They distort reality to serve their own ends, manipulating others through charm or ruthless aggression. These hugely damaging individuals can be difficult to dislodge but HR should help to manage them out of the business wherever possible. They are not coachable and will not change. The explosive bully Fortunately, many workplace bullies are capable of change. This includes the large category whose aggressive behaviour results from low emotional intelligence and the failure to contain negative, blaming feelings when under stress.

Let's look at Jacqui, an example of bullying that many HR directors will recognise. One of four directors on the executive committee of a financial services business, Jacqui was highly conscientious, with a track record of meeting her targets. HR advised she receive coaching when complaints about her behaviour from team members and fellow directors came to a head. While Jacqui's style was naturally quite controlling, she was respected for her technical abilities and for getting things done. When she felt pressured however, especially when her performance was in the spotlight in the run-up to Board presentations, she would micro-manage her colleagues, chasing them before deadlines were due and double-checking their work. Even minor errors or setbacks would trigger furious outbursts. She would attack the colleagues concerned, whether subordinate or peers, accusing them of incompetence or carelessness in blistering terms. On some occasions staff were reduced to tears and one direct report had been signed off with stress. The business decided to act after receiving a deputation from several of those on the receiving end of Jacqui's undermining and intimidating behaviour.

As this illustrates, explosive bullies cause great pain to others. Yet, like Jacqui, they are often high-performers who identify strongly with their organisations, possess at least some capacity to empathise and do not set out to hurt. It's important for HR to understand their behaviour. Psychologically, the key lies in their need to feel competent and in control. Outwardly confident, they are often inwardly insecure and over-dependent on external recognition. These individuals are extremely task-focused, with high standards and a powerful drive to achieve, and they invest great emotional energy in their work. While this combination of qualities often leads to external success, it can also fuel unacceptable behaviour within their organisation. Executives such as Jacqui suffer from a kind of 'inner tyrant' - a critical internal voice that continually exhorts them to achieve and succeed. The threat of failure - for example a mistake by a subordinate on whose work they depend - triggers painful anxiety and shame. Feeling under attack, the leader automatically responds with a defensive fight reaction. As adrenaline floods their body, they experience a surge of anger. Blame for the problem is allocated to others who then experience the sense of inadequacy which the bully is trying to escape.

The inner tyrant has become the outer tyrant. Tackling the problem When challenged, the explosive bully is usually defensive, denying their behaviour or placing the responsibility on others. They reject the accusation of bullying and often feel furious that the organisation to which they feel they give so much is attacking them. Difficult as it is, HR and senior stakeholders must ride out these objections. They must describe the unacceptable behaviour, emphasising the weight of evidence gathered from all those affected, insist on change and spell out the consequences of failure. Once this message - repeated as necessary - has been successfully delivered, the bully should be offered intensive specialist coaching, usually with 360-degree feedback, on a non-negotiable basis. Progress should be carefully monitored with improved behaviour affirmed and poor behaviour immediately re-addressed. HR has a vital role to play in this process.

Those organisations who find the courage and skill to put a stop to explosive bullying reap a huge return on their investment. Not only will the morale and performance of staff be transformed but the former bully will also raise their contribution to a new level.

Here's an example by the Manitoba Government in Canada, as to not what to do!!

And for the first female security officer hired at Selkirk Mental Health Centre in Manitoba, Canada a forensic psychiatric unit is no place not to get feedback from one's supervisor: [7]

> *SHMC Union Representative Requested for my Probation Review Board 19th January, 2011?*
> *Sent: December 31, 2010 5:52:18 AM*
> *To: L. Bob (HEALTH) (bob.l@gov.mb.ca)*
> *Cc: resourcecentre@mgeu.ca*
> *Bcc: debbie.k@gov.mb.ca*
>
> *Re: Wednesday 29th December meeting*
> *Re: Official Request for a Union Rep*
>
> *Bob L*
> *Manager, Security Services*
> *Selkirk Mental Health Centre*
> *Phone: (204) 482-1606*
> *Fax: (204) 785-8936*
> *Email: bob.l@gov.mb.ca*
>
> *Hi Bob,*
>
> *Further to your meeting with me on December 29th, 2010 during which:*
>
> *You gave me a "heads-up" that there had been a few minor complaints during my six months' probation period (July 19, 2010 to January 19, 2011);*
>
> *That you wanted me to make my probation and that the complaints apparently consisted of:*
>
> *a) C.D. apparently complained that I was not searching the male patients – however, I was following your instructions in your e-mail dated 18th October 2010 that it was SHMC policy that only "same sex" searches be done ["current policy dictates that the search to be performed by a same sex staff member – male for male – female for female – it can be witnessed by a staff member of either sex"];*

As C.D. is apparently being groomed for the supervisor position, C.D. should know the Center's policy about "same sex" searches – so why has he complained about me following the Center's policy?

The only time "opposite sex" searches are allowed according to your further e-mail is during an emergency.

b) C.D. apparently complained that during slow periods I was using a simple pen and paper notepad to edit a story I have been working on?

However C.D. has never apparently complained about other security who use their personal laptops to watch movies, etc during their shifts?

Also apparently C.D. has not complained about one particular security who apparently sleeps quite a bit during his "graveyard" shift?

c) C.D. also apparently indicated that I do not get on with the other security?

I would like proof of this, as I work well with the other security and staff [PNAs and nurses] on all the units, and I willingly perform any duty that the other security direct me to do.

In fact, on several occasions staff [PNAs and nurses] in other units have expressed surprise that I have come into their units while I am on my patrol(s) to see how things are going and to make a security presence known – many saying they rarely see security staff come into their unit during the evenings.

The only other security staff member who gave me "static" was S.F. who kept insisting that I search male patients irrespective of the Center's policy of "same sex" searches – and I believed that he complained to C.D. about this – so C.D. should have put an end to S.F.'s insistence that I breach SHMC "same sex" search policy – but apparently C.D. did not do that – and apparently made the same complaint to you?

Why C.D. would do that makes no sense, especially as he is apparently in line for the supervisor spot.

This doesn't help our security department's consistency in being in line with SHMC patient policy, including visitor searches.

d) I'm aware that several PNAs and nurses have complained about the "sexist comments" that some of the security make while in the control room.

I must ask, does C.D. feel uncomfortable with me being a female security officer?

Would C.D. prefer an <u>all-male</u> security force at SHMC [an "old boys'" club]?

As a potential supervisor, it's always nice to be upfront with your "crew" so that they can learn and not just complain behind their back – as apparently C.D. has done in complaining to you without being given the benefit of his experience at SHMC.

It would have been nice had he approached me to explain the problem(s) as far as he saw my apparent error(s).

e) *Finally, on another note, apparently I scored the lowest on the Sheriff's training – however, that's not surprising since I was the only female in the course.*

The fact remains that I <u>passed</u> the Sheriff's training and was awarded the "Certificate of Completion" by the Sheriff instructors.

I spoke with a Union Rep [Sandy Young, switchboard operator] at SHMC last night 30 December 2010 about your meeting with me on 29th December, 2010 who said:

I should have had a Union Representative with me during your meeting with me on Wednesday 29th December, 2010;

She also gave the impression that the (minor) complaints were "nit-picking", and that she was under the impression that our security officer training was inconsistent, which might explain the reason for these?

As such, I am making a formal request that:

I be represented by a Union Representative regarding and during my probation review board;

That if available Tim Byers [ext. 697, Area 7] who has apparently been a long time Union Rep at SHMC be approached to represent me as my Union member;

If Tim is unavailable I am putting in a request to my Union today [MGEU] that they help me identify a Union Representative at SHMC to represent me during my probation review;

My preference would be a long-time <u>female</u> Union Rep if possible.

I also request:

My Union Rep and I meet with you <u>before</u> my probation review board on 19th January 2011 so my Union Rep can be given details of the <u>minor</u> complaints you mentioned on 29th December, 2010, including <u>when</u> the complaints were made, <u>who</u> made the *complaints, and any other <u>pertinent</u> information my Union Rep would need to represent me at my probation review board;*

That the meeting with you, my Union Rep, and myself occur significantly <u>before </u>my probation review date of 19th January 2011 so that my Union Rep will have time to digest the information prior to, and be able to prepare for, my actual probation review board;

That my Union Rep as well as myself be informed of the <u>actual</u> <u>date/time/location </u>of my probation review board.

In closing, I would like to add:

I have <u>always </u>turned up for my shifts, usually a good half hour beforehand;

I have <u>never</u> missed a shift;

I have <u>always</u> come at a "moment's notice" when you called me because someone had called in sick at the last minute or were unable to do their shift for some reason;

I have <u>always</u> been glad to help SHMC and you out;

I have given 100% to my job and have enjoyed every minute of it;

I hope I pass my probation review board as I wish to make SHMC a long term career goal.

Finally, did you still want me to do the fill-in 14th January, 2011 shift [1700 to 0100 hrs] for the security officer that wanted this shift off?

Thank you very much,

The first female security officer at SMHC

cc. SMHC Union Rep requested
MGEU, <u>resourcecentre@mgeu.ca</u>

cc. Debbie Ky HR Rep
SHMC, <u>debbie.k@gov.mb.ca</u>[8]

This email also went unanswered by her supervisor, as did several other emails go unanswered by her supervisor [B.L.], together with this one:[9]

I believe my belonging & room searches are correct - please advise otherwise?
Sent: January 13, 2011 8:01:23 AM
To: L, Bob (HEALTH) (bob.l@gov.mb.ca)
Cc: debbie.k@gov.mb.ca
Bcc: timothyebyers@hotmail.com; bod-area5@mgeu.ca

13 January, 2011

Bob L
Manager, Security Services
Selkirk Mental Health Centre
Phone: (204) 482-1606
Fax: (204) 785-8936
Email: bob.l@gov.mb.ca

cc. Danah B, CEO
Debbie K HR Consultant
SMHC, debbie.k@gov.mb.ca

cc. Tim Byers, MGEU -SMHC Union Rep
timothyebyers@hotmail.com
bod-area5@mgeu.ca

Hi Bob,

On the advice of my Union rep following my 11 January 2011 meeting with the CEO, he advised to cc copies to all concerned.

The reason I write today is that the CEO during my 11 January meeting mentioned:

Are you searching the rooms also', with respect to my being a 'team-player' indicating that this aspect is also something the other security officers have complained about.

The CEO also questioned if 'you search the bags and personal belongings' of guests and visitors.

This is the first I've heard of these complaints.

Isn't an employee supposed to hear about complaints at the time they happen?

My reply to this information from the CEO is this:

I have been taught by the other security officers the general procedure with respect to body-searching is for one [same sex] security guard and one of the staff [usual a PNA] to attend to the patient or guest.

Usually the PNA is the individual whom at this particular point in time will search any of the patient's/visitors' personal belongings - bags while the person is getting body-searched by a [same sex] security officer.

If there are a number of patients to be searched and there are additional security officers around they may go and assist the original officer do body searches [if the same sex] otherwise they can do belonging - bag searches, which I always do to assist my fellow SOs.

The only time I couldn't assist in doing belongings - bags searches [and this applies to my male SO counterparts] is when there is only two security officers on duty and one has to be in the control room [as per policy] – in these situations the same sex SO leaves the control room and does the body searches, while the PNAs do the belonging – bag searches.

So, I don't see where the complaint is being made that I am not a team player and that I do not search belongings and bags?

I might also add that I have never skirted my responsibilities, including my fair share of room searches.

What I have even proposed to <u>all</u> the male SOs is that, if they have males to search, to 'even out the work' I will do the room searches.

This, however, has obviously not appeased those male SOs that do not want me on site because I cannot do male searched.

If this is not correct procedure, please advise.

In fact, if truth be told – I've been the brunt of double duty when it comes to some of these same male SOs that do not want me on site because I cannot search males.

For example, on December 30th, 2010 one of the PNAs [C.] was annoyed that, although I had just returned to Area 15 after a 2 ½ hour patrol, the other male SO who had sat in the control room for those 2 ½ hours immediately told me to do a room search.

What appears to be the case is that the same male SOs who have clearly indicated they do not want me on site because I cannot search male patients / visitors have <u>embellished their complaints</u> about this [you revealed their male search complaints *on 29 December 2010] with the above 'revelation' that I am not searching belongings or rooms, which is not the case whatsoever!*

J.Mat. [spelling?] on 08 January 2011:
 "Why is she coming in";
"She can't do anything";
"I have to do the searches" (i.e., the male searches).
"We don't want any female SO on the weekend as they cannot do the work" (i.e., search male patients / visitors).

C.D. [spelling?] still gives me the "cold shoulder" because I am not searching male patients / visitors.

S.F. [spelling?] recently protested on 12 December 2010 that I was not searching male patients and even held everyone up because he had to email Bob L right away to complain, while the PNAs were 'demanding' he hurry up with his email to Bob L.

B.S. [spelling?] recently said to me that "if I couldn't do male searches than why bother (doing the job)".

Thanks

The first female security officer hired at SMHC[10]

As cited by Poole & Regoli (1980), "while numerous findings emerged from the study, the most general showed that as a prison guard's work relations with inmates, fellow officers, and administrators deteriorate, his level of cynicism increases."[11]

And what could cause more cynicism but a supervisor that refuses to reply to a security officers' emails in a maximum security forensic unit, as this B.L. refused to reply to the first female security officer hired at SMHC.[12]

The RCMP seemed to be no better. As cited, "the Mounties want you to believe they take sexual harassment allegations seriously. But when you listen to Janet Merlo's story, the RCMP's oft-repeated declaration rings hollow."[13]

"In September, 2007, Constable Merlo wrote to then-RCMP commissioner William Elliott … Ms. Merlo waited for a reply. And waited. Until one day it finally arrived – more than two years later."[14]

"In November, 2009, she received a letter from deputy commissioner Peter Martin, writing on behalf of his boss. It began by thanking Ms. Merlo for 'your correspondence of Aug. 19, 2007,' and referenced her allegations of harassment."[15]

"As you are aware the RCMP does not take these allegations lightly and, in fact, has an obligation to provide a harassment free environment for all of our employees," he wrote.[16]

"Janet Merlo didn't know whether to laugh or cry."[17]

"I couldn't believe it," said Ms. Merlo, who retired from the force last year. "I couldn't believe the gall of them writing back to me more than two years after the fact. And then saying they took my claims seriously. As far as I'm concerned, that told me everything you need to know about how serious the RCMP takes harassment on the job and what kind of priority it is."[18]

As asked in the course 700 Intro to Safety Management[19], "are policies based on objective, factual information, or subjective hunches?"[20]

Stating further, "policies based on hunches occur most often in fear-driven corporate cultures."[21]

Obviously, the RCMP apparently falls into this category:

> *"I know for a fact there are at least six women that I know [who] have left the force or are still in that have suffered harassment," Carle said. "I'm sure there are others who are afraid to come forward for fear of reprisals."[22]*

As further noted, "sexual harassment of women thrives in environments that are male dominated, hierarchal and demand strict adherence to codes of silence like the RCMP," said MacDougall, noting female officers are afraid to speak up.[23]

Benson-Podolchuk has also accused RCMP of trying to obtain confidential medical information from her doctor, pulling her over during a highway traffic stop for no reason and threatening "consequences" if she didn't quit.[24]

"She says the abuse left her afraid to go to work, embarrassed, intimidated and afraid for her personal safety."[25]

As mentioned in the course 700 Intro to Safety Management[26], the RCMP have apparently adopted a managerial approach of "threat of punishment" where their "culture is fear-driven."[27]

Here are some examples of what a tough-coercive leader might say:
Punishment - "If I go down...I'm taking you all with me!"
Punishment - "If you report hazards, you will be labeled a complainer."[28]

Another point relates to communication. As cited, "the most basic communication theory talks about the requirement for both a sender and receiver in the communication process ... The sender initiates the communication and the receiver receives, interprets, and responds to the communication."[29]

"Where and how the process ends depends on the purpose of the communication and the dynamics of the process itself. Even the simplest communication between two individuals may be a very complicated process."[30]

With respect to the first female security officer hired at the Selkirk Mental Health Centre in Manitoba, Canada maybe the requests of the supervisor [B.L.] were too complicated for him to understand, as he replied to none of the officers email communications?[31]

Here's another email that went unanswered by the supervisor [B.L.]?[32]

important to clarify if C.D. an unofficial supervisor?
Sent: January 17, 2011 2:06:54 AM
To: L, Bob (HEALTH) (bob.l@gov.mb.ca)
Cc: danah.b@gov.mb.ca
Bcc: bod-area5@mgeu.ca; resourcecentre@mgeu.ca

17 January, 2011

Bob L
Manager, Security Services
Selkirk Mental Health Centre
Phone: (204) 482-1606
Fax: (204) 785-8936
Email: bob.l@gov.mb.ca

cc. Danah B,
Chief Executive Officer
Selkirk Mental Health Centre
Box 9600, Selkirk, Manitoba R1A 2B5
Phone: 204 482-1607
Danah.B@gov.mb.ca

cc. Tim Byers, MGEU -SMHC Union Rep
timothyebyers@hotmail.com
bod-area5@mgeu.ca

cc. The Equity and Human Rights Committee
MGEU Head Office, resourcecentre@mgeu.ca

Hi Bob,

First let me say that any queries I had about my 11 January 2011 meeting with the CEO should be cc'd to those involved, according to my Union rep who was also at the meeting.

As such, maybe you can answer this.

During my meeting with CEO Danah B on 11 January 2011 she indicated that C.D. was not the supervisor nor was he being groomed for supervisor?

If this is the case, why is C.D. giving 'tests' to security as if he were the supervisor?

Have you given him permission to act as supervisor and give 'tests' to security?

If not, then why did C.D. leave a message in our Communication Log Book and dated 14 January 2011 the first day I worked last week:

C.D. wrote words to the effect that he had 'tested' S.F., and C.D. found that S.F. was the best 'standard' for security at SMHC'.

[It should be noted that someone tried to white out the author of the message, but if you look at the back it appears to be C.D.'s name as the author]

[It should also be noted there has never been a message like this in our log book before]

What was the purpose of this message in our Communication Log Book?

Was it one 'old time' <u>guard</u> supporting another 'old time' <u>guard</u>?

Aren't C.D. and S.F. 'left-overs' from the old security firm [CORS] that supplied security <u>guards</u> for SMHC?

Isn't C.D. one of the male security at SMHC that doesn't want me on site because I cannot search male patients / visitors [even though he knows full well that SMHC has a 'same sex' search policy and I cannot search males as per your email dated 18 October 2010]?

Isn't this sex discrimination under the Code?

Isn't C.D. the guy that complained that I am not a team player because I do not search male patients / visitors although I cannot under SMHC's 'same sex' search policy?

Likewise, isn't S.F. one of the male security that doesn't want me on site because I cannot search male patients / visitors?

Again, isn't this sex discrimination under the Code?

Wasn't it S.F. who just had to email you on 12 December 2010 protesting that I was not searching male patients / visitors and even held everyone up from doing our work while he emailed you?

Even the PNAs were 'demanding' S.F. hurry up with his email to you so we could finish our work [even though S.F. knew full well that SMHC has a 'same sex' search policy and I cannot search males as per your email dated 18 October 2010]?

The question is, was the CEO mistaken during my 11 January 2011 meeting and you've actually given C.D. permission to be a supervisor?

If not, it's unfortunate C.D. feels himself to be a supervisor because these two 'old time' guards have apparently inflamed other new male SOs [hired during my competition and even the competition after mine] with their same 'hang-ups' or apparent 'sexist' attitude.

For example, B.S. has adopted their 'old <u>guard</u>' attitude and doesn't want me on site because I cannot search male patients / visitors.

B.S. recently said to me that "if I couldn't do male searches than why bother (doing the job)".

Again, isn't this sex discrimination under the Code?

Similarly, when Jeremey Matovich heard I was coming in on 08 January 2011 to fill a 'sick' shift, he told another SO: "Why is she coming in"; "She can't do anything"; "I have to do the searches" (i.e., the male searches); "We don't want any female SO on the weekend as they cannot do the work" (i.e., search male patients / visitors).

Again, isn't this sex discrimination under the Code?

Sort of bolsters my impression that SMHC should have cleaned-house when they went to in-house Security <u>Officers</u> [a much more professional category, where some are more 'in tune' with a respectful work environment, and the 'new' standards expected of employees toward each other and to clients (patients) as per the Code and out of decent courtesy].

Thanks for a reply to clarify if C.D. is a 'supervisor' and, if not, why is he 'testing' other security and placing the info in our Communication Log Book [which wasn't intended for such 'personal' messages]?

Thank you,

The first female security officer hired at SMHC[33]

The email doesn't seem that complicated, however, the supervisor failed the first tenant of a manager – "provide feedback in a timely manner? Aren't you ignoring them? Again, it's the worst of all possible responses."[34]

And a forensic psychiatric unit is a most dangerous place.[35]

An interesting development in this case occurred when the Selkirk Mental Health Centre included documentation about discrimination / fair treatment of other employees, although denying the first female security officer hired at SMHC had been treated unfairly[36] [see Appendix 1a, 1b and 1c cited below]?

Footnotes

1 - 2. *700 Intro to Safety Management*
Steven J. Geigle, MA, CET, CSHM
OSHAcademy Safety and Health Training
www.oshatrain.org

3. *Walking amongst the cannibals! Watching out for the sharks?*
http://www.amazon.com/Walking-amongst-cannibals-Watching-sharks/dp/146647291X/ref=sr_1_30?s=books&ie=UTF8&qid=1320314090&sr=1-30

See also: *Black Balled by Manitoba Government for making sex-discrimination complaint*
http://www.amazon.com/BLACK-BALLED-Manitoba-Government-sex-discrimination/dp/1466480890/ref=sr_1_32?s=books&ie=UTF8&qid=1320313966&sr=1-32

4 – 6. *Perverts, Sexual Deviants Occupy Top RCMP Ranks – New Allegations Suggest*
Saturday, November 12th, 2011
http://thelinkpaper.ca/?p=11604

7 - 10. *Walking amongst the cannibals! Watching out for the sharks?*
http://www.amazon.com/Walking-amongst-cannibals-Watching-sharks/dp/146647291X/ref=sr_1_30?s=books&ie=UTF8&qid=1320314090&sr=1-30

11. Eric D. Poole & Robert M. Regoli, "Work Relations and Cynicism Among Prison Guards", *Criminal Justice and Behavior*, September 1980, Volume 7(3), pp. 303 – 314.

12. *Walking amongst the cannibals! Watching out for the sharks?*
http://www.amazon.com/Walking-amongst-cannibals-Watching-sharks/dp/146647291X/ref=sr_1_30?s=books&ie=UTF8&qid=1320314090&sr=1-30

13 - 18. *RCMP took two years to respond to officer's sexual harassment complaint*
Gary Mason, Last updated Friday, Jan. 06, 2012
http://m.theglobeandmail.com/news/national/british-columbia/gary_mason/rcmp-took-two-years-to-respond-to-officers-sexual-harassment-complaint/article2261049/?service=mobile

19 - 21. *700 Intro to Safety Management*
Steven J. Geigle, MA, CET, CSHM
OSHAcademy Safety and Health Training
www.oshatrain.org

22. *Perverts, Sexual Deviants Occupy Top RCMP Ranks – New Allegations Suggest*
Saturday, November 12th, 2011
http://thelinkpaper.ca/?p=11604

23. *Female RCMP officers' accounts of sexual harassment in force prompt new hotline*

By Suzanne Fournier, The Province November 25, 2011
http://www.theprovince.com/news/Female+RCMP+officers+accounts+sexual+harassment+force+prompt+hotline/5763916/story.html

24 - 25. *Manitoba Mountie Files Sexual Harassment Suit*
Regina Leader-Post, RCMP Watch: Who is keeping them accountable?
http://webcache.googleusercontent.com/search?q=cache:eC7AV88HMxEJ:www.rcmpwatch.com/manitoba-mountie-files-sexual-harassment-suit/+RCMP+Const.+Nancy+Sulz+wins+a+%24950,000+lawsuit&cd=1&hl=en&ct=clnk&gl=ca

26 - 30. *700 Intro to Safety Management*
Steven J. Geigle, MA, CET, CSHM
OSHAcademy Safety and Health Training
www.oshatrain.org

31 - 33. *Walking amongst the cannibals! Watching out for the sharks?*
http://www.amazon.com/Walking-amongst-cannibals-Watching-sharks/dp/146647291X/ref=sr_1_30?s=books&ie=UTF8&qid=1320314090&sr=1-30

34. *700 Intro to Safety Management*
Steven J. Geigle, MA, CET, CSHM
OSHAcademy Safety and Health Training
www.oshatrain.org

Also see: *"Managers cause accidents; they just cause them in different ways than workers and supervisors. However many layers there are in an organization we can see a causal connection back to the accident. Presidents cause accidents. They can fail to lead, to set policy, to ensure a proper delegation of authority, to inspire a proper safety culture, to design a workable organizational structure or to allocate resources."*
Reference to *The Internal Responsibility System*
By: Dr. Peter Strahlendorf
2001-03-01
http://www.ohscanada.com/news/the-internal-responsibility-system/1000156181/

35. Robert L. Sadoff. *Ethical Issues in Forensic Psychiatry: Minimizing Harm*. John Wiley, 2011.

36. *Conspiracy? Manitoba government style?*
http://www.amazon.com/Conspiracy-Manitoba-government-Terry-Mallenby/dp/1468142070/ref=sr_1_52?s=books&ie=UTF8&qid=1325503212&sr=1-52

Appendix 1a

Also note: *As the author of Conspiracy? Manitoba government style? asked, if there wasn't anything to the first female security officer hired at Selkirk Mental Health Centre sex-discrimination / unequal treatment complaint to the Manitoba Human Rights Commission file # 11 EN 027, then why was this pamphlet being given out with staff pay stubs?*

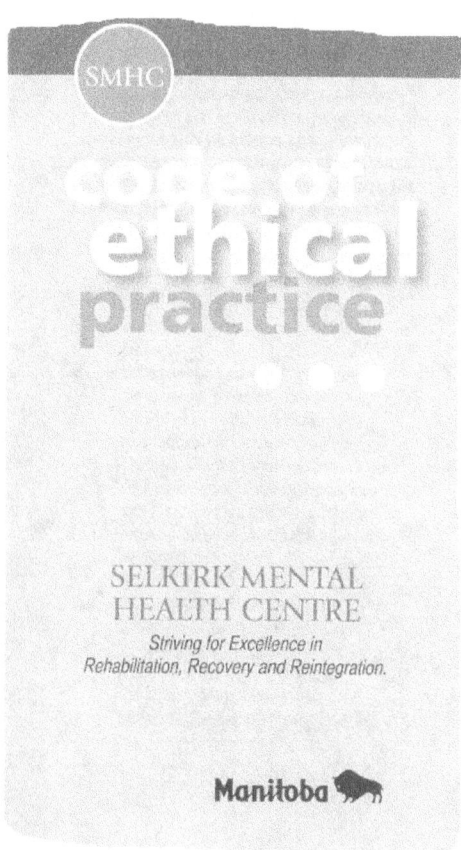

Reference: *Conspiracy? Manitoba government style?*
http://www.amazon.com/Conspiracy-Manitoba-government-Terry-Mallenby/dp/1468142070/ref=sr_1_52?s=books&ie=UTF8&qid=1325503212&sr=1-52

"Managers cause accidents; they just cause them in different ways than workers and supervisors. However many layers there are in an organization we can see a causal connection back to the accident. Presidents cause accidents. They can fail to lead, to set policy, to ensure a proper delegation of authority, to inspire a proper safety culture, to design a workable organizational structure or to allocate resources."
Reference to *The Internal Responsibility System*
By: Dr. Peter Strahlendorf

2001-03-01
http://www.ohscanada.com/news/the-internal-responsibility-system/1000156181/

Appendix 1b

Also note: *As the author of Conspiracy? Manitoba government style? asked, if there wasn't anything to the first female security officer hired at Selkirk Mental Health Centre sex-discrimination / unequal treatment complaint to the Manitoba Human Rights Commission file # 11 EN 027, then why was this pamphlet being given out with staff pay stubs?*

Section 4
Personal and Professional Conduct

4.1   **Respect** – Staff/Associates shall respect the dignity and individuality of all persons. A respectful workplace values courteous conduct, positive communication, mutual respect and collaborative working relationships (See General Policy A-03).

4.2   **Abuse** – Staff/Associates must ensure that patients, staff and associates are provided with a safe and secure environment, free of abuse and harassment (See General Policies E08-01 – E08-15)

Reference: *Conspiracy? Manitoba government style?*
http://www.amazon.com/Conspiracy-Manitoba-government-Terry-Mallenby/dp/1468142070/ref=sr_1_52?s=books&ie=UTF8&qid=1325503212&sr=1-52

"Managers cause accidents; they just cause them in different ways than workers and supervisors. However many layers there are in an organization we can see a causal connection back to the accident. Presidents cause accidents. They can fail to lead, to set policy, to ensure a proper delegation of authority, to inspire a proper safety culture, to design a workable organizational structure or to allocate resources."
Reference to *The Internal Responsibility System*
By: Dr. Peter Strahlendorf
2001-03-01

http://www.ohscanada.com/news/the-internal-responsibility-system/1000156181/
Appendix 1c

Also note: *As the author of Conspiracy? Manitoba government style? asked, if there wasn't anything to the first female security officer hired at Selkirk Mental Health Centre sex-discrimination / unequal treatment complaint to the Manitoba Human Rights Commission file # 11 EN 027, then why was this pamphlet being given out with staff pay stubs?*

Section 5
Breach of the Code

If you have any reasonable suspicion that a Staff or Associate has violated The Code, you have an obligation to report this to the Area/Service supervisor. Supervisors are responsible for gathering the facts and consulting with Human Resources regarding their findings. Violations of The Code could result in disciplinary action being taken, up to and including termination of employment or other contractual relationship.

Reference: *Conspiracy? Manitoba government style?*
http://www.amazon.com/Conspiracy-Manitoba-government-Terry-Mallenby/dp/1468142070/ref=sr_1_52?s=books&ie=UTF8&qid=1325503212&sr=1-52

"Managers cause accidents; they just cause them in different ways than workers and supervisors. However many layers there are in an organization we can see a causal connection back to the accident. Presidents cause accidents. They can fail to lead, to set policy, to ensure a proper delegation of authority, to inspire a proper safety culture, to design a workable organizational structure or to allocate resources."
Reference to *The Internal Responsibility System*
By: Dr. Peter Strahlendorf
2001-03-01
http://www.ohscanada.com/news/the-internal-responsibility-system/1000156181/

Chapter 3 - System approaches to safety

In the course 700 Intro to Safety Management[1] it is emphasized that:

"Accidents are part of a broad group of events that adversely affect the completion of a task. These events are incidents. For simplicity, the procedures discussed in this course apply most appropriately to accidents, but they are also applicable to all incidents in general. Think of it this way: accidents cause injuries and incidents do not." [1]

Proper supervision and procedures are a key feature to prevent unwanted incidents that result in staff accidents. The supervision at the Selkirk Mental Health Centre, as cited in previous chapters, appeared to fall well short of this mark.[3]

Accidents, as cited, can include:

"Struck-by. A person is forcefully struck by an object. The force of contact is provided by the object.

Struck-against. A person forcefully strikes an object. The person provides the force or energy.

Caught-on. A person or part of his/her clothing or equipment is caught on an object that is either moving or stationary. This may cause the person to lose his/her balance and fall, be pulled into a machine, or suffer some other harm.

Caught-in. A person or part of him/her is trapped, or otherwise caught in an opening or enclosure.

Caught-between. A person is crushed, pinched or otherwise caught between a moving and a stationary object, or between two moving objects.

Fall-To-surface. A person slips or trips and falls to the surface he/she is standing or walking on.

Fall-To-below. A person slips or trips and falls to a level below the one he/she was walking or standing on.

Over-exertion. A person over-extends or strains himself/herself while performing work.

Bodily reaction. Caused solely from stress imposed by free movement of the body or assumption of a strained or unnatural body position. A leading source of injury.

Over-exposure. Over a period of time, a person is exposed to harmful energy (noise, heat), lack of energy (cold), or substances (toxic chemicals/atmospheres).

Contact-by. Contact by a substance or material that, by its very nature, is harmful and causes injury.

Contact-with. A person comes in contact with a harmful substance or material. The person initiates the contact."[4]

There are many examples of each:

Struck-by Accidents

As mentioned:

"*Struck-by accidents are those where an object hits the worker. These accidents are frequently related to material handling and housekeeping. Poorly stacked material may fall or slide. Objects blocking aisles could cause bumps or tripping. Overhead storage shelves, racks, hangers, aisles, passageways, and doors can be a source of danger. Careless work habits can make hazards worse. Struck-by accidents can also occur during tree trimming, pruning, and felling. The tree or tree limbs can fall and strike workers on the ground or in the tree. Bent limbs can also strike workers when the limb is released and springs back.*"[5]

An example:

"*A faller was standing on the narrow ledge of a cliff to buck a windfall tree. The windfall's rootwad was lying on the perimeter of the ledge and was only loosely attached to the ground. Most of the windfall's 58-foot trunk was suspended between two standing trees below the ledge. As the faller completed the bucking cuts, the rootwad rolled downhill off the ledge, causing the lower part of the trunk to pivot on one of the standing trees. Then as the suspended trunk swung uphill, its bucked end pinned the faller against the cliff. He sustained fatal injuries.*"[6]

Struck-against Accidents

As noted:

"*According to the Bureau of Labor Statistics, about 150,000 construction accidents occur every year in the United States. The Occupational Safety and Health Administration, meanwhile says one in ten construction workers are injured in the US annually.*"[7]

In their study, Santos *et. al.* (2010) "More than one-half of the injuries sustained were sprains and strains … Other injuries were also reported (e.g., concussion, cuts, lacerations, puncture, joint inflammation); however, each of these only accounted for less than 2 percent of the total injuries."[8]

And, "the most frequently injured body part was the back (N=221, 36%), followed by multiple body parts (N=137, 22%), the neck (N=82, 13%), and shoulder(s) (N=43, 7%). Injuries to other body parts were also reported; however, each of these accounted for less than 4 percent of the total injuries."[9]

An example of falling against an object, in this case an unprotected blade:

"On July 13, 2000, Employee #1, of Senor Felix Gourmet Mexican Food, Inc., was using a horizontal mixer to make salsa. There was no visible model or serial number on the mixer unit itself; however, according to the quality assurance manager the make was Reitz S.S. ribbon blender, model #RS 24-20, serial #10162." [10]

"Employee #1 was standing in front of the discharge gate. After emptying the salsa from the mixer into the bin, he was reaching with his left hand to press the STOP button of the mixer when he slipped."[11]

"As he slipped, his right hand entered the discharge gate, amputating his thumb and index finger. The plant manager took him first to Foothill Medical Center, then to Intercommunity Hospital, and finally to the Western Hand Center."[12]

"According to Employee #1 and coworkers, the front guard on the discharge gate was not in place at the time of the accident."[13]

"During a visit by OSHA on July 17, 2000, the floor of the salsa mixing area was wet. The physical, environmental, and human factors that contributed to this accident were (1) failure to have in place the guard for the discharge gates; (2) the presence of wet, slippery floors; and (3) failure to identify during the quarterly inspection that the guard was missing."[14]

Caught-on Accidents / Caught-in Accidents / Caught-between Accidents

An example of "caught-on" accident was reported:

"On 3/11/92, in Raleigh, NC a rigger was hooking up steel beams onto a "Christmas tree lift with bullchokers;" where the crane hook was hooked to one main (longer) load line with several cable slings attached at intervals below the crane hook. The "bullchoker" attachments to the main line were covered by a metal reinforcing "bull-ring." The rigger had hooked up the first two beams of the Christmas tree lift and went to hook up a third one while the first two were being raised by the crane. The second beam got caught on the "bull-ring" of the lower attachment on the main cable causing the beam to slip off and fall across the rigger's legs."[15]

In another "caught-on" accident involved:

"A young worker was cutting 3/8-inch board with a skill saw. His glove caught on the edge of the board and the saw lacerated his arm."[16]

This raises an important point that young workers a more prone to accident, injury or death on work-sites. As cited:

"A recent report from the National Institute for Occupational Safety and Health (NIOSH) shows that workers 24 and younger are twice as likely to suffer workplace injuries and wrongful death as other workers."[17]

"Among the most common were injuries resulting from construction accidents, such as being struck by or caught in industrial equipment. Construction was also the industry with the second highest rate of fatal accidents."[18]

"The report was an analysis of on-the-job injuries and deaths occurring between 1998 and 2007. Overall, nearly 8 million young workers were injured, with the highest rate of accidents among workers who were 18 and 19."[19]

"The most common types of accident for all workers, but particularly for young people, were being struck by or against a tool or machine, being rubbed or abraded, or being caught in or crushed in machinery."[20]

An example of "caught-in" accident was reported:

"A Moncks Corner man died Tuesday morning at a Summerville plant after he became entangled in a cement auger while performing maintenance on the machine. Lamar Ravenell, 48, died at a local hospital from traumatic injuries, Berkeley County Coroner Bill Salisbury said. He said the incident happened about 11 a.m. at Sanders Brothers asphalt plant, just off U.S. Highway 17A. Salisbury said Ravenell was doing maintenance when he became caught in the machine. He was cut loose by firefighters and taken to a local hospital where he later died. The death was ruled accidental, Salisbury said."[21]

Another young worker example included:

"A young worker's coveralls were caught in the shaft of the lead pulley on a running conveyor."[22]

An example of "caught-between" accident was reported:

"On Wednesday, February 22, a female dockworker was killed at Port Newark, New Jersey, in an industrial accident. The 47-year-old dockworker was unloading a container ship at a Newark port at the time of the accident. She tragically became caught between railroad car-sized metal containers that had been removed from a ship in Newark Bay. The crushing injuries that resulted ultimately proved to be fatal."[23]

"Sadly, the injured dockworker was pronounced dead by physicians at University Hospital at 8:34pm. Prior to her passing, she was a member of the International Longshoreman's Association, a maritime worker union. The container terminal where her fatal accident occurred was privately run. It is located near Tyler and Mohawk Streets in Newark's East Ward. An investigation has been launched into the circumstances of the woman's death. Authorities have also notified the federal Occupational Safety and Health Administration about the tragedy."[24]

Another young worker example included:

"Beamsville, ON-based Admiral Welding & Mfg. Inc. has been fined $40,000 for a violation of the Occupational Health and Safety Act in which a young worker was injured."[25]

"In May 2009, a co-op student was using a brake press to bend a large piece of steel. His hands became caught between the upper and lower dies of the press, causing injuries. The brake press lacked a guard to prevent access to the pinch point between the dies."[26]

"Admiral Welding & Mfg. Inc. pleaded guilty to failing to ensure that any part of a machine that may endanger the safety of any worker shall be equipped with and guarded by a guard or other device that prevents access to the pinch point, a violation of O. Reg. 851, section 25."[27]

How many situations can be prevented?

As cited in the course 700 Intro to Safety Management:

"We like to think that accidents are unexpected or unplanned events, but sometimes, that's not necessarily so. Some accidents result from hazardous conditions and unsafe behaviors that have been ignored or tolerated for weeks, months, or even years. In such cases, it's not a question of "if" the accident is going to happen: It's only a matter of "when." But unfortunately, the decision is made to take the risk."[28]

Continuing, let's look at examples of Fall-To-surface / Fall-To-below accidents.

Fall-To-surface Accidents / Fall-To-below Accidents

As outlined:

"Falls from elevation hazards are present at most every jobsite, and many workers are exposed to these hazards daily. As such, falls are an important topic for occupational safety and health services. Any walking/working surface could be a potential fall hazard. An unprotected side or edge which is 6 feet or more above a lower level should be protected from falling by the use of a guard rail system, safety net system, or personal fall arrest system."[29]

"These hazardous exposures exist in many forms, and can be as seemingly innocuous as changing a light bulb from a step ladder to something as high-risk as installing bolts on high steel at 200 feet in the air. Falls are the second leading cause of work-related deaths in the U.S.[2] In 2000, 717 workers died of injuries caused by falls from ladders, scaffolds, buildings, or other elevations."[30]

"Companies must make sure that they follow the applicable safety legislation (e.g. the Occupational Safety and Health Act in the United States) in order to keep the work environment safe."[31]

As further noted:

"According to the 2009 data from the Bureau of Labor Statistics, 605 workers were killed and an estimated 212,760 workers were seriously injured by falls to the same or lower level. The highest frequency of fall-related fatalities was experienced by the construction industry, while the highest counts of nonfatal fall injuries continue to be associated with the health services and the wholesale and retail industries."[32]

As further reported:

"Once the third leading cause of work-related death across all industries, falls have surpassed workplace homicide to become the second leading cause after motor vehicle crashes. Last year alone, some 717 workers died of injuries caused by falls from ladders, scaffolds, buildings, or other elevations. That equaled almost two deaths per day on average."[33]

"In the construction industry, falls lead all other causes of occupational death, but the risk is present in virtually every kind of workplace."[34]

An example of a "fall" accident was reported:

"A 60-foot plummet killed a Redcliff man on a construction site Thursday afternoon."[35]

Police say the 33-year-old construction worker was at or near the top of a "taller, industrial type of building" around 4 p.m. when he fell.[36]

"It is not known exactly what happened but this incident is not seen as suspicious."[37]

"The investigation is still ongoing; given the place and the circumstances Occupational Health and Safety have been called in and they're going to be conducting a full investigation into exactly what caused this to happen," said Acting Cpl. Mike Martin of the Redcliff RCMP.[38]

In another "fall" accident it was reported:

"Searchers found a sweater and hard hat Friday near the spot where a painter plunged from the Throgs Neck Bridge in New York City. The Throgs Neck, a suspension bridge, connects Queens and the Bronx at the point where the East River meets Long Island Sound."[39]

"Authorities said several hours after John Massas, 35, fell 140 feet that he was almost certainly dead, the New York Daily News reported. Police and the U.S. Coast Guard began a search using helicopters and boats soon after the 8:05 a.m. accident."[40]

"It's recovery at this point," a source told the newspaper.[41]

"By early afternoon, the searchers had discovered the sweater and hard hat floating."[42]

"Massas, a member of the International Union of Painters and Allied Trades, was part of a 15-man crew working on the Throgs Neck Bridge. It was his second day on the job."[43]

Maria Rosso, the local union's office manager, called him a "nice regular guy working hard to make a living." She said he lived in the Bronx with his wife and daughter and was hoping to move to New Jersey.[44]

"El Sol Contracting & Construction Corp., the contractor on the repainting job, was cited in 2007 after one of its employees was killed by a fall from the Verrazano Narrows Bridge."[45]

As cited in the course 700 Intro to Safety Management, under the New Theory - Systems Approach:

"A competent person can examine workplace conditions, behaviors and underlying systems to predict closely what kind of accidents will occur in the workplace."[46]

"The systems approach takes into account the dynamics of systems that interact within the overall safety program."[47]

"It concludes that accidents are considered defects in the system. People are only one part of a complex system composed of many complicated processes (more than we realize). Accidents are the result of multiple causes or defects in the system. It becomes the investigator's job to uncover the root causes (defects) in the system."[48]

"Fixing the system, not the blame, is the heart of the investigation."[49]

"To prevent accidents, the system must work more safely."[50]

As further cited elsewhere[51], a critical element of an OHSMS is the implementation phase. This includes:

- *"Allocation of appropriate resources (personnel & equipment);*
- *Defining & communicating OHS responsibilities & accountabilities;*
- *Training of employees in relation to safe systems/ processes;*
- *Ensuring employee effective consultation & communication with employees/stakeholders;*
- *Proactively controlling workplace risks;*
- *Managing contractor OHS exposures; and*
- *Establishing capability to deal with a range of emergency situations."*[52]

As further stated[53], knowledge of line personnel is particularly important at this stage. For example, by including:

- *"OHS training in existing training frameworks & programs.*
- *OHS clauses into existing contractor tender specifications and contracts.*
- *OHS responsibilities and accountabilities into existing position descriptions and performance review processes.*
- *Risk assessments in job scheduling and planning."*[54]

Naturally your safety system has to be continually evaluated and, as mentioned, this will include:

"Having implemented the system, the measurement and evaluation stage checks that the system is operating effectively."[55]

"Activities include workplace inspections, testing of equipment (e.g. machine guards), incident management and auditing."[56]

"Having an OHSMS helps to capture findings from incident investigations and inspections and improve systems."[57]

Another approach to workplace safety includes "the internal responsibility system, or IRS, is a system in which every individual is responsible for health and safety."[58]

As mentioned:

"It can be thought of as your organizational chart, with a clear set of statements about responsibility and authority for health and safety listed for each person -- no exceptions."[59]

"Accountability is built right into the organizational structure."[60]

"Second, the people in this hierarchical structure interact with each other to identify and solve health and safety problems and to seek opportunities to improve the processes they are involved with."[61]

"Everyone at all levels takes initiative on health and safety. As well, everyone is obligated to report unresolved concerns upward and to respond properly to the unresolved concerns of others."[62]

Footnotes

1 - 2. *702 Accident Investigation*
Steven J. Geigle, MA, CET, CSHM
OSHAcademy Safety and Health Training
www.oshatrain.org

3. Reference: *Conspiracy? Manitoba government style?*
http://www.amazon.com/Conspiracy-Manitoba-government-Terry-Mallenby/dp/1468142070/ref=sr_1_52?s=books&ie=UTF8&qid=1325503212&sr=1-52

4. *702 Accident Investigation*
Steven J. Geigle, MA, CET, CSHM
OSHAcademy Safety and Health Training
www.oshatrain.org

5. *Struck-By Accidents for Trainers and Supervisors*
Keith L. Smith, Associate Vice President for Agricultural Administration and Director, Ohio State University Extension, The Ohio State University
https://docs.google.com/viewer?a=v&q=cache:WAEuhV6ETToJ:ohioline.osu.edu/aex-fact/192/pdf/0192_2_74.pdf+accident+Struck-by&hl=en&gl=ca&pid=bl&srcid=ADGEEShNKent6IY_-Qaf5whoGAzOZ0Vovow7WYb613pQ2nDoNYJmfZRXXBW0D__lqCuEqGCXAi-kjpw5R_SOyknv5KZhOUCmv5_ispHeeS26-sWZI9TiYeRkuIn2bdEBKeyJpO5b-TOI&sig=AHIEtbQMjJ9lyoaLnyB9mPp6iy4tmPXQtg

6. *Investigation Reports - Primary Resources: Faller dies when struck by bucked tree*
http://www2.worksafebc.com/Topics/AccidentInvestigations/IR-PrimaryResources.asp?reportID=35759

7. *Top 6 Facts about Construction Accidents*
http://www.infobarrel.com/Top_6_Facts_about_Construction_Accidents

8 – 9. Brenda R. Santos, William L. Porter, Alan G. Mayton. *An Analysis of Injuries to Haul Truck Operators in the U.S. Mining Industry: Struck Against Moving Object*, National Institute for Occupational Safety and Health, Office of Mine Safety & Health Research also see Proceedings of the Human Factors and Ergonomics Society Annual Meeting September 2010 vol. 54 no. 21 1870-1874
https://docs.google.com/viewer?a=v&q=cache:fgKaXhGXyXEJ:www.cdc.gov/niosh/mining/pubs/pdfs/aaoit.pdf+Accidents+%22Struck-

against&hl=en&gl=ca&pid=bl&srcid=ADGEESg2YR0f0d89cjLPS656OJv_W1LVE8ry
y8Rt0cgP8MFJ8Y1tfNu_TRk6zOj12HGbETNHRCaetNMVIg_FKGJptIIEekBeLt2mJX
9pDU1Kx0k3smEFskjfzP5gxVkoQRRi_dbmuBJl&sig=AHIEtbQfu5oliTjE6H9KqR3V
GF9x5v6ktA

10 – 14. *Accident Details And Descriptions: Accident: 120331954 - Finger Amputated In Ribbon Mixer*
David Matheny, 2003-2005
http://vegaslawyer.net/Amputated.html

15. *OSHA Archive Document*
MEMORANDUM FOR: John B. Miles Jr., Regional Administrator Region I
FROM: Charles Culver, Director, Office of Construction and Engineering
SUBJECT: Christmas Treeing
September 9, 1993
OSHA Archive Document
http://www.osha.gov/pls/oshaweb/owadisp.show_document?p_id=21256&p_table=INTE
RPRETATIONS

16. 2006 *Incidents Involving Young Workers*
Injury Type : Lacerated arm
Core Activity : Framing
Location : Central Interior
ID Number : 2006143950322
Date of Incident : 2006-Nov
WorkSafeBC (the Workers' Compensation Board of BC)
http://www2.worksafebc.com/Topics/YoungWorker/WCBInitiatives-
YWAccidents.asp?reportid=34455

17 - 20. *Young Workers Twice as Prone to Workplace & Construction Accidents*
Johnston, Moore & Thompson.
http://www.huntsvillepersonalinjurylaw.com/2010/07/young-workers-twice-as-prone-to-
workplace-construction-accidents.shtml

21. *SC worker killed after getting caught in machine*
From staff reports - postandcourier.com
http://www.heraldonline.com/2012/03/06/3798717/worker-killed-after-getting-
caught.html

22. *Incidents Involving Young Workers*
Injury Type : Abrasion and bruising of leg
Core Activity : Manufacture of concrete products
Location : Lower Mainland
ID Number : 2006117670145
Date of Incident : 2006-Nov

WorkSafeBC (the Workers' Compensation Board of BC)
http://www2.worksafebc.com/Topics/YoungWorker/WCBInitiatives-YWAccidents.asp?reportid=34455

23 – 24. *Maritime Accident News: Female Dockworker Killed in Tragic New Jersey Maritime Fatality*
Posted on Mar 12, 2012
Vujasinovic & Beckcom P.L.L.C
http://www.maritimeaccidentattorney.com/news/female-dockworker-killed-in-tragic-new-jersey-maritime-fatality-20120312.cfm

25 – 27. *In the Courts: Brake press injures co-op student*
Ontario Ministry of Labour
http://www.iapa.ca/main/apmag/in_the_courts.aspx

28. *702 Accident Investigation*
Steven J. Geigle, MA, CET, CSHM
OSHAcademy Safety and Health Training
www.oshatrain.org

29 – 31. *Falling (accident)*
http://en.wikipedia.org/wiki/Falling_(accident)

32. *Fall Injuries Prevention in the Workplace*
Centers for Disease Control and Prevention -
The National Institute for Occupational Safety and Health (NIOSH)
http://www.cdc.gov/niosh/topics/falls/

33 – 34. *STRATEGIC PRECAUTIONS AGAINST FATAL FALLS ON THE JOB ARE RECOMMENDED BY NIOSH*
Centers for Disease Control and Prevention -
The National Institute for Occupational Safety and Health (NIOSH)
http://www.cdc.gov/niosh/updates/fatalfal.html

35 – 38. *Construction worker dies in fall*
Damien Wood, Calgary Sun
First posted: Friday, August 05, 2011 04:01 PM MDT
http://www.calgarysun.com/2011/08/05/construction-worker-dies-in-fall

39 – 45. *U.S. News: Worker killed in fall from bridge*
Published: March. 30, 2012 at 3:00 PM
http://www.upi.com/Top_News/US/2012/03/30/Worker-killed-in-fall-from-bridge/UPI-80351333134038/

46 – 50. *702 Accident Investigation*

Steven J. Geigle, MA, CET, CSHM
OSHAcademy Safety and Health Training
www.oshatrain.org

51 – 56. *Health and Safety Risk Management: Systems Approach to Managing Safety*
by Riskex on May 20, 2010
in Safety Systems
http://www.safetyrisk.com.au/2010/05/20/systems-approach-to-managing-safety/

58 – 62. *The Internal Responsibility System*
By: Dr. Peter Strahlendorf
2001-03-01
http://www.ohscanada.com/news/the-internal-responsibility-system/1000156181/

Chapter 4 – Accident court cases

It's important to review some court cases dealing with employee accidents to appreciate the requirements imposed on employers, and the consequences should they fall short of their responsibility in guaranteeing a safe work environment for their employees.

Struck by court case

In this case, "the Defendant (Westfair) plead guilty that, on or about May 3, 2001, it did, being an employer at a place of employment, fail to make arrangements for the transport and handling of plants and trolleys in a manner that protects the health and safety of workers, contrary to section 12(b) of the Occupational Health and Safety Regulations, 1996, of Saskatchewan."[1]

The facts of the accident included:

"[6]   The employee who was injured, Ava Malisiewicz, had been an employee of Westfair, since age 16, for approximately 10 years at the time of the accident. About 6 weeks earlier she had been promoted to the position of Supervisor of the Home and Garden Department.

[7]   On the morning of May 3, 2001 a delivery truck, operated by a Milner Greenhouses employee, arrived at the rear dock of the Superstore with a delivery of plants and flowers. The driver was told to drive around to the front to unload the truck. He was very new to the job and this was his second solo delivery. The truck was rented and equipped with a power lift gate with which he was unfamiliar. He had received no training in safe operating procedures.

[8]   The driver asked for the assistance of Ms. Malisiewicz. He rolled a rack of plants and flowers on to the power lift gate and while holding the rack with his hands to steady it, attempted to lower the lift gate by reaching for the operating control with his right foot. As he tapped on the operating control with his foot, the rack became unsteady and it fell forward off the lift gate, onto Ms. Malisiewicz. She had been standing on the ground, several feet below and directly in front of the rack with arms outreached in an attempt to steady it.

[9]   Ms. Malisiewicz received emergency services at the scene and was taken to hospital where she underwent extensive surgery. She suffered a collapsed lung and damage to her ribs and vertebrae. As a result of the damage to her spinal chord she was paralysed from the waist down."[2]

The liability stemmed from the fact that the employer only implemented proper procedures after the accident:

"[11]   Westfair had not made suitable arrangements for the safe delivery of the plants. Nor had it provided adequate training to its employee about the risks of assisting in the unloading of plants. Westfair had not provided written safe work procedures. These were developed after the accident."

"[15]   Following the accident Westfair immediately put a new procedure into place for unloading plants. It undertook a formal hazard analysis of all job functions in the Home and Garden Department and developed and by March 2002 had implemented a written operations and safety manual for use in its Leisure and Home and Garden Department, in all Superstores. The new receiving procedure was outlined in the Westfair brief (paragraph 37):

(a) The driver must notify the Department Supervisor or Store Manager that a plant order has arrived. He may not unload any racks without supervision by a Department Supervisor or Store Manager;

(b) The Department Supervisor or Store Manager must set up a safety zone with caution cones ten feet back from the end deck of the truck. This person is responsible for ensuring that no one enters the safety zone;

(c) The driver is responsible for unloading the rack and pushing it through the safety zone where store staff will check off the items and roll them to the Garden Centre for unloading. Once the plant racks have been unloaded or if produce is being refused and returned to Milner Green houses, it is the driver's responsibility to reload the empty racks or the racks containing refused product. The reloading is supervised by the Store Manager or Supervisor with the same safety zone set up and enforcement."[3]

In its reasoning, this Court examined the responsibility of the employer under their respective OHS regulations:

"[19]   I will begin with pertinent provisions of The Occupational Health and Safety Act, 1993 and The Occupational Health and Safety Regulations, 1996. Westfair plead guilty to a charge of failing to comply with section 12(b) of the Occupational Health and Safety Regulations, 1996, found under Part III General Duties. Section 12 provides:

General duties of employers

12 The duties of an employer at a place of employment include:

(a) the provision and maintenance of plant, systems of work and working environments that ensure, as far as is reasonably practicable, the health, safety and welfare at work of the employer's workers;

(b) arrangements for the use, handling, storage and transport of articles and substances in a manner that protects the health and safety of workers;

(c) the provision of any information, instruction, training and supervision that is necessary to protect the health and safety of workers at work; and

(d) the provision and maintenance of a safe means of entrance to and exit from the place of employment and all worksites and work-related areas in or on the place of employment."[4]

Section 3 also included:

"3 Every employer shall:

(a) ensure, insofar as is reasonably practicable, the health, safety and welfare at work of all of the employer's workers;

(b) consult and co-operate with any occupational health committee or the occupational health and safety representative at the place of employment for the purpose of resolving concerns on matters of health, safety and welfare at work;

(c) ensure, insofar as is reasonably practicable, that the employer's workers are not exposed to harassment at the place of employment;

(d) co-operate with any other person exercising a duty imposed by this Act or the regulations; and

(e) comply with this Act and the regulations."[5]

The Court also listed Section 13:

"Section 13 of the Act and section 22 of the Regulations, address the duty to provide occupational health and safety programs, referred to in the Report of the Occupational Health Officer. They provide:

13(1) An employer at a prescribed place of employment shall establish and maintain an occupational health and safety program or a prescribed part of an occupational health and safety program in accordance with the regulations.

(2) An occupational health and safety program must be established and designed in consultation with:

(a) the occupational health committee;

(b) the occupational health and safety representative; or

(c) the workers, where there is no occupational health committee and no occupational health and safety representative.

(3) An occupational health and safety program must include all documents, information and matters that are prescribed in the regulations.

(4) An occupational health and safety program must be in writing and must be made available to the occupational health committee, the occupational health and safety representative, the workers or an occupational health officer on request.

(5) Where the work at a place of employment is carried on pursuant to contracts between a contractor and two or more employers, the contractor shall co-ordinate the occupational health and safety programs of all employers at the place of employment."[6]

As well as Section 22:

"22(1) Subject to subsection (2), an occupational health and safety program required by section 13 of the Act must include:

(a) a statement of the employer's policy with respect to the protection and maintenance of the health and safety of the workers;

(b) the identification of existing and potential risks to the health or safety of workers at the place of employment and the measures, including procedures to respond to an emergency, that will be taken to reduce, eliminate or control those risks;

(c) the identification of internal and external resources, including personnel and equipment, that may be required to respond to an emergency;

(d) a statement of the responsibilities of the employer, the supervisors and the workers;

(e) a schedule for the regular inspection of the place of employment and of work processes and procedures;

(f) a plan for the control of any biological or chemical substance handled, used, stored, produced or disposed of at the place of employment and, where appropriate, the monitoring of the work environment;

(g) a plan for training workers and supervisors in safe work practices and procedures, including any procedures, plans, policies or programs that the employer is required to develop pursuant to the Act or any regulations made pursuant to the Act that apply to the work of the workers and supervisors;

(h) a procedure for the investigation of accidents, dangerous occurrences and refusals to work pursuant to section 23 of the Act at the place of employment;

(i) a strategy for worker participation in occupational health and safety activities, including audit inspections and investigations of accidents, dangerous occurrences and refusals to work pursuant to section 23 of the Act; and

(j) a procedure to review and, where necessary, revise the occupational health and safety program at specified intervals that are not greater than three years and whenever there is a change of circumstances that may affect the health or safety of workers."[7]

When considering what consequences this employer would suffer, the Court referred to:

"[33]   When one examines Part IX of the Occupational Health and Safety Act, Offences and Penalties, sections 57 and 58, it is evident that not all offences under the Act are to be treated with equal gravity. Generally the maximum fine increases with the apparent gravity of the offence. The Defendant has plead guilty to contravening a regulation having regard to an incident which resulted in the serious injury of an employee. The maximum fine available for that same contravention increases with the seriousness of the outcome or consequences. The amount of the potential fine in this Part is affected by whether the particular offence causes or is likely to cause death or serious injury. The maximum fine also increases with, the number of offences, in the event that the offence is continuing in nature, and for second or subsequent offences. Two of the offences enumerated in section 57 require intention and a third addresses the failure to comply with an order, decision or direction made pursuant to the Act or Regulations, and these latter three offences are grouped together with the respect to the potential penalty.

[34]   In this case as the contravention was associated with serious injury, the maximum fine is $300,000. Where an individual is convicted of a contravention that caused serious injury or death, he or she is also liable to a term of imprisonment of up to 2 years. Intention or knowledge is not a specific element of the offence for which this Defendant was charged, however it carries the greatest penalty available under the Act."[8]

NOTE: An employer that is responsible for all third parties coming onto their premises that may cause [in part or in-whole] injury to its employees

The Court also made it clear that it is the employer that is responsible for all third parties coming onto their premises that may cause [in part or in-whole] injury to its employees:

"[42]   This discussion goes to the very purpose of occupational health and safety legislation and the requirement that the employer make arrangements to keep the work environment safe for its employees. This responsibility requires that, whatever the practices of third parties, that an employer make responsible arrangements for the safety of its employees that serve to anticipate and respond to potential risks, including those risks posed by third parties."[9]

Finding:

"[43] The risk was foreseeable. Ms. Malisciewicz's former supervisor, who trained her, informed investigators that she was not aware of a formal training program or orientation for safe work procedures with respect to the delivery of plants. Ms. Malisciewicz felt that her training was rushed and that a lot was thrown at her all at once. She had witnessed her supervisors assist in the delivery of plants in the same fashion at least twice and was not provided with any verbal instruction or information pertaining to safety. The Occupational Health Officer wrote in her report that at the time of the incident there was no written safe work procedure(s) in place and that past practice was that the vendor unloaded product with assistance from workers employed in the home and garden department. Independent of the responsibility of Milner Greenhouses, Westfair failed to meet its responsibility to provide a safe work environment when it had the ability to do so, both with respect to its contractual arrangements with Milner Greenhouses and its instruction to employees in the Home and Garden Department."[10]

The fine imposed:

"[52] I find that a fine in the sum of $30,000, is appropriate having regard to the importance, primarily, of general deterrence. In this context I have considered: the apparent size, sophistication, and financial resources of the Defendant, the failure to have any safety procedures in place in the Home and Garden Department, notwithstanding the foreseeability of the danger, the seriousness of the injury, the range of fines in this jurisdiction, and the maximum fine available."[11]

Another fall accident court case

This case involve a fall, and the attempts of the worker to obtain a disability pension.

As cited:

"[12]   *On December 27, 1983, while in the process of hooking up an empty pallet dolly to a tractor, the worker slipped on an ice covered steel pallet that was on the ground. The worker landed on his buttocks, mainly on the left side of his sacrum and on his left arm. The worker finished his shift and also started work the next day, but had to log off due to pain in his buttocks and left hip. After leaving work on December 28, 1983, the worker attended at a local walk-in clinic where he was examined by Dr. I. Scarborough. Dr. Scarborough had x-rays taken and diagnosed a soft tissue injury.*

[13]   The worker was not satisfied with Dr. Scarborough's diagnosis – he felt that the examination was inadequate and sought the opinion of Dr. W. Rothman, a chiropractor. Dr. Rothman reviewed the worker's x-rays and concluded that the worker had dislocated his coccyx.

[14]   After the Christmas holiday, the worker returned to work and attended at the OHS and was seen by Dr. Tucker on January 5, 1984. On examination, the worker complained of "severe discomfort on attempting to walk or move his left hip." The worker identified his left sacroiliac joint and the muscles just below the joint as the site of his discomfort, as well as discomfort on attempting to move the hip. Dr. Tucker described the incident as follows: "fell on Dec 26 on his buttocks – mainly on left side of sacrum & left arm when his feet gave out from under him. Worked next day but then had to lay off because of pain in buttocks and left hip."

[15]   Dr. Tucker examined the worker and noted extreme pain with palpation of the coccyx as well as soft tissue swelling. Dr. Tucker diagnosed a dislocation of the coccyx, as well as soft tissue sprain. Dr. Tucker asked the worker to bring in his x-rays on his next visit. Dr. Lee, also a chiropractor, provided the worker with a note dated January 4, 1984, which stated that the worker had dislocated his coccyx, sprained his sacroiliac and thus was unable to work."[12]

As cited at paragraph 6, the worker was denied a permanent disability assessment and a permanent disability ("PD") award for a low back injury resulting from a December 27, 1983, workplace accident.[13]

The issue on appeal was, as cited at paragraph 8, "… is whether the worker is entitled to a PD award arising out of the December 27, 1983, work-related incident."[14]

As noted at paragraph 9 and 10, "the worker is 47 years old" and "… was hired as an airport station attendant by the employer, an airline."[15]

In a following incident, the court note:

"*[21]   On August 31, 1987, the worker, while grooming a cabin, crouched between two rows of seats to reach refuse under the seats – the worker felt the sudden onset of severe pain in his lower back. The worker went to OHS and was examined by Dr. Wright. The worker related the pain to his fall in 1984. He advised Dr. Wright he had broken his coccyx and that following the break a dull ache was always present, and after a double shift he felt stabs of pain in the lumbar region L2-L3. The worker further reported that after the accident, he had been to a specialist who advised that he had a back problem and needed to do exercises. The worker was diagnosed with back strain and remained off of work in the care of his family physician, Dr. Dworak. In his physician's first report Dr. Dworak noted that the worker strained his back five years ago when he fell on the tarmac.*"[16]

Another incident included:

"*[23]   On November 9, 1988, the worker was bent over, cleaning between the seats on an aircraft when he experienced strain and muscle seizure in his lower back. The worker sat down until the pressure eased. Dr. Dworak described the injury as back pain and spasm of the lumbar spine and diagnosed the worker with a recurrence of a September 1987 injury. The worker underwent an x-ray of his lumbar spine on November 10, 1988. The worker's vertebral bodies and intervertebral discs were intact and normal, and both his sacroiliac joints were well maintained.*"[17]

In terms of the OHS department, they concluded the x-rays were 'essentially negative examinations'.

"*[27]   In an evaluation dated October 19, 1989, Dr. R. Evans, a doctor with the OHS office, listed the worker as a Class II station attendant with permanent restrictions for heavy physical effort, frequent bending or stooping and lifting heavy weights over 10 kilograms.*

[28]   On June 18, 1992, the worker had x-rays taken of his lumbar spine and coccyx. In the opinion of Dr. McIntyre, radiologist, the lumbar spine demonstrated no abnormality. With respect to the worker's sacrum and coccyx, Dr. McIntyre identified anterior angulation of the distal coccygeal segments but did not find an obvious cause. Dr. McIntyre opined that the angulation of the worker's distal coccygeal segments was "a congenital variation" and found "no evidence of recent trauma…."

[30]   On August 11, 1994, the worker had x-rays taken of his lumbar spine, pelvis and coccyx. In the opinion of Dr. McIntyre, radiologist who read

the worker's June 18, 1992 x-rays, the lumbar spine, pelvis and hips demonstrated no abnormality, the sacrum and coccyx were intact, and the anterior angulation of the distal coccygeal segments was likely a variation of normal. In sum, the x-rays were 'essentially negative examinations' ...

[39]   In a joint statement dated September 22, 1999, two of the worker's colleagues confirmed that they had personal knowledge of the worker's December 26, 1983, lower back accident and his constant pain and discomfort since that time. The co-workers further attested that they "went to his rescue" on numerous occasions during their own shifts due to the "painful affliction" that limits the worker's movements.

[40]   The worker was seen again by Dr. Naumetz on December 10, 1999. Dr. Naumetz noted that the worker was seen about his chronic low back pain. Dr. Nautmetz stated that:

[b]asically he has claims with the Workplace Safety and Insurance Board...due to a fall on the tarmac while working for [the accident employer] on December 26, 1983. He claims to have injured his back. He also has [another claim] which refers to another episode of acute back pain on March 4, 1998. Apparently these claims are not being recognized by [the Board]. I am not clear why this is. He, however, would like to apply for a type of disability pension. I have looked at previous films from Milton dating back to 1998 and these show a reasonably normal appearing lumbar spine but there is an anterior tilt of the sacrum at the sacrococcylgeal junction, which could relate to an old fall. He has pain in the paraspinal muscles of the low lumbar region, as well as the buttocks, and the pains will also radiate down into the legs."[18]

However, in the next OHS department exam it was noted:

"[33]   On April 3, 1998, the worker again had x-rays taken of his lumbar spine, sacrum and coccyx. In the opinion of Dr. McIntryre, the radiologist who read the worker's August 11, 1994, x-rays, the lumbar spine demonstrated no abnormality, however, he also opined that "[t]he sacrum and coccyx show significant anterior displacement of the coccygeal segments of the lower spine. There is also some displacement of the segments so that this may well be a traumatic displacement and represent a recent fracture."[19]

Followed with:

"[36]   At the behest of the claims adjudicator, on August 18, 1998, a field investigation was undertaken. The field investigator spoke with the worker, the employer's WSIB specialist and a co-worker. The worker described being in constant pain since the December 26, 1983 injury. The WSIB specialist confirmed that the worker was on a list of permanently disabled employees and had been so for a long time. The co-worker described the worker complaining a lot about his back between 1984 and 1985

and in 1989 when the cabin services division was dissolved. Additionally, the co-worker advised that for the past six to seven years he had not worked with the worker, but did see him about once a month. The co-worker described the worker's then current job as "...involving a lot of sitting at a desk, but that he seems to be tolerating it.

[37]   *According to the OHS' clinical notes, on August 31, 1998, the worker attended at the OHS office for a medical review at the recommendation of a supervisor. The clinical notes state that:*

[the worker] has chronic disability that is self-established on the basis of his level of activation. Reports chronic myofascial back pain since 1983. Attributes situation to fall onto buttocks 1983. Has had assessment by consultant orthopaedic surgery. Dx mechanical back pain. Does have facet involvement L5-S1. Zero surgical lesion. Established with permanent partial disability Oct 1989....Reports that the constant sitting is problematic. This is causing him to be more symptomatic with lumbar back pain. He finds some relief with activity/mobility...A – Chronic myofascial lumbar pain."[20]

However, a medical consultant for OHS determined, as cited at paragraph 50, "… in a memorandum dated October 12, 2004, Dr. Garg opined that there did not appear to be a permanent impairment resulting from the 1983 incident. Further, Dr. Garg opined that neither the sclerotic changes at L1 nor the coccydynia resulting from the fracture evident on the April 3, 1998, x-ray were compensable."[21]

The court also cited the pertinent law and policy:

"[71]   The worker claims a permanent disability arising out of a December 27, 1983, work-related accident, as such any entitlement would be governed by the Workers' Compensation Act, R.S.O. 1980 (the "pre-1985 Act") as amended by the Workplace Safety and Insurance Act, 1997 ("WSIA").

[72]   Pursuant to section 43(1) of the pre-1985 Act:

Where permanent disability results from the injury, the impairment of earning capacity of the worker shall be estimated from the nature and degree of the injury, and the compensation shall be a weekly or other periodical payment during the lifetime of the worker, or such other period as the Board may fix, of a sum proportionate to such impairment not exceeding in any case the like proportion of 75 per cent of his average weekly earnings during the twelve months immediately preceding the accident or such lesser period as he has been employed."[22]

NOTE: Definitive medical evidence is required for a permanent disability pension, specifically related to a given back injury

In concluding, the court found:

"[75]   There is no question that the worker has chronic, episodic back pain. There is also no question that the December 26, 1983, workplace accident was serious. However, the Panel is not convinced that the December 26, 1983, incident resulted in a permanent impairment of the worker's lower back.

[76]   Having reviewed all of the medical evidence, what is clear to the Panel is that, contrary to his testimony, the worker's back problems pre-date the December 26, 1983, workplace accident. As noted in the OHS clinical notes, on January 25, 1983, some twelve months prior to the December 26, 1983, incident, the worker sought care from the OHS office. At this time, the worker complained of a two year history of intermittent back pain, which had recently worsened. The worker reported no history of trauma, but related his symptoms to the nature of his employment, specifically bending and lifting."[23]

As such, the court held:

"[74]   In the view of the Panel the evidence does not support the worker's claim that he suffered a permanent disability as a result of the December 26, 1983, workplace incident ...

[87]   The Panel is not persuaded that the worker suffered a permanent impairment as a result of the December 26, 1983, incident."[24]

With a disposition of, "the appeal is denied."[25]

Another fall prevention court case

This court case was about OHS regulations about scaffolding and portable ladder(s) on work sites.

As cited:

"[3]   On February 15, 2011 this officer did an inspection in the Town of Lunenburg where the restoration work for the Bluenose 11 is underway. As a result of the inspection the officer issued 6 warnings and 2 orders, as follows:

Warning(1) OH&S Act. 38-1-b Availability of information at workplace.

Warning(2) A current telephone number for reporting OHS concerns to the Division.

Warning(3) MSD sheets shall be kept updated every 3 years.

Warning(4) Employer and Employees shall use fall protection as required by the Regulations.

Warning(5) Employers and Employees will use a fall arrest system and have attached to an anchor point, worn at all times.

Warning(6) Occupational Safety General Regulations 23-1 Emergency Showers and eyewashes.

Order #1131810007-001 Employer shall ensure that mental scaffolding is erected maintained and dismantled in accordance with manufacture's specifications, must be complied with by February 22, 2011. This order resulted in Administrative Penalty and was appealed by the Appellant.

Order #1131810007-002 Employer shall ensure that any portable ladder used on site has a firm footing and is secured in an adequate manner against movement. Employer will hold a safety talk with employees on the site to stress the importance of ladder safety. This order was complied with on February 25, 2011."[26]

As cited elsewhere:

"Lunenburg - The Bluenose ll, Nova Scotia's sailing ambassador has been attracting attention worldwide since work on its restoration began in Lunenburg. Web cams have attracted people from as far away as Kuwait."[27]

"In May 2009, the provincial and federal government announced support for a major restoration of the Bluenose II. The project is valued at $14.8 million."[28]

"In July 2010, the province of Nova Scotia awarded a $12.5 million contract for the restoration of Bluenose II to a consortium of three Nova Scotia shipyards."[29]

Continuing the court case, the main question to be answered involved:

"Order #1131810007-001 Employer shall ensure that mental scaffolding is erected maintained and dismantled in accordence with manufacture's specifications, must be complied with by February 22, 2011. This order resulted in Administrative Penalty and was appealed by the Appellant."[30]

NOTE: OHS violations will lead to Administrative Penalties at the least

In determining this issue, the court cited the OHS regulation in paragraphs 6 and 7:

"[6]   Section 4(1) of the OHS Administrative Penalties Regulations provides that "the Administrator may require a person who has contravened a provision of the Act or its regulations to pay an administrative penalty by serving a notice of administrative penalty on the person."

[7]   The amount set for an administrative penalty, the factors which may lead to its adjustment, and the circumstances in which a penalty should be doubled are set out in Section 5, 6 & 7 of the OHS Administrative Penalties Regulations."[31]

On looking at the administrative penalty, the court cited that:

"[8]   The base amount of an administrative penalty is determined in accordance with the table set out in Section 5 of the OHS Administrative Penalties Regulations. The table indicates different administrative penalty amounts depending on the "Class of Person" who contravened the Occupational Health and Safety Act of Nova Scotia or its regulations, and whether or not the contravention resulted in injury or had the potential to result in immediate injury.

[9]   In the Notice of Administrative Penalty, the Administrator determined that the "Type of Workplace Party" was an Employer. The Administrator also determined that the contravention could not have resulted in an injury or had potential to result in immediate injury. As such, the Administrator determined that the base amount of $500.00 in Column 'A' of Section 5 of the OHS Administrative Penalties Regulations was applicable."[32]

And, at paragraph 12, recorded:

"[12]   I have reviewed the records considered by the Administrator as well as the submissions and evidence from the Appellant and Director and find that the base amount of $500.00 is appropriate in this case."[33]

The court noted when an administrative penalty could be adjusred:

"[13]   Section 6 (1) and (2) of the OHS Administrative Penalties Regulations provides as follows:
(1)   The Administrator may increase or decrease the administrative penalty in Section 5 based on the following factors:

(a)   the efforts to prevent the contravention from occurring;

(b)   whether or not the person on whom the administrative penalty is imposed derives an economic benefit from the contravention;

(c)   the harm the contravention causes to any person.

(2)   Unless the administrative penalty is doubled under Section7, the maximum administrative penalty that may be imposed is as set out in the following table…"[34]

With the court finding:

"[25]   In view of the factors in Section 6 of the OHS Administrative Penalties Regulations, I find that the base penalty amount of $500.00 should be adjusted to $400.00.

[30]   In conclusion, the decision of the Board on the Administrative Penalty in question is as follows: Administrative Penalty #1131810007-001 is confirmed in the amount of $400.00."[35]

One reason for this decision, as emphasized by the employer at paragraph 4:

"[4]   In its submission, the Appellant argues that: (1) No injury or harm occurred; (2) All workers had fall protection training; (3) All workers were wearing fall arrest protection; (4) All workers attended regular hazard assessment meetings regarding fall protection; (5) The area of hazard in question was corrected immediately upon notification of a potential hazard by a supervisor; (6) Our company has no previous penalties or convictions; (7) Our company holds regular tool box meetings for all workers; and (8) Our company has a full time JOSH Committee which reports to management."[36]

Footnotes

1 - 11. *R. v. Westfair Foods Ltd., 2005 SKPC 26 (CanLII)*
Date: 2005-04-27
Docket: 31550250
Parallel citations: [2005] 10 WWR 752; 263 Sask R 162

http://www.canlii.org/eliisa/highlight.do?text=fined+not+Securing+accident+scene&lang
uage=en&searchTitle=Search+all+CanLII+Databases&path=/en/sk/skpc/doc/2005/2005s
kpc26/2005skpc26.html

12 - 25. *Decision No. 2405/07, 2008 ONWSIAT 809 (CanLII)*
Date: 2008-03-26
Docket: 2405/07
http://www.canlii.org/eliisa/highlight.do?text=OHS+Fall+accident+&language=en&searc
hTitle=Search+all+CanLII+Databases&path=/en/on/onwsiat/doc/2008/2008onwsiat809/2
008onwsiat809.html

26. *Lunenburg Shipyard Alliance Limited (Re), 2012 NSLB 3 (CanLII)*
Date: 2012-01-03
Docket: OHS-0365
http://www.canlii.org/eliisa/highlight.do?text=ohs+fines&language=en&searchTitle=Sear
ch+all+CanLII+Databases&path=/en/ns/nslb/doc/2012/2012nslb3/2012nslb3.html

27 - 29. *Bluenose ll restoration attracts global audience*
By Kevin Jess
Feb 11, 2011
http://digitaljournal.com/article/303548

30 - 36. *Lunenburg Shipyard Alliance Limited (Re), 2012 NSLB 3 (CanLII)*
Date: 2012-01-03
Docket: OHS-0365
http://www.canlii.org/eliisa/highlight.do?text=ohs+fines&language=en&searchTitle=Sear
ch+all+CanLII+Databases&path=/en/ns/nslb/doc/2012/2012nslb3/2012nslb3.html

Chapter 5 - Securing the accident scene

In the course 700 Intro to Safety Management[1] it is emphasized that:

In any accident that is reportable (serious or fatal) injury might trigger an OSHA accident investigation, where, "at the request of OSHA, the employer must mark for identification, materials, tools or equipment necessary to the proper investigation of an accident."[2]

It is also important that material evidence does not somehow get lost or "walk off" the scene.[3]

As further mentioned, two things may disappear after an accident occurs:

"Material evidence - Material evidence is anything that might be important in helping us find out what happened. Somehow, tools, equipment, and other items just seem to move. The employer is anxious to 'clean up' the accident scene so that people can get back to work. It's important to develop a procedure to protect material evidence so that it does not get moved or disappear. If evidence disappears, I'm sure you can see why it might be difficult to uncover the surface causes for the accident. If you can't uncover the surface causes, it will be almost impossible to discover and correct the root causes. We'll talk more about surface and root causes later in the course."[4]

"Memory - Accidents are traumatic events that result in both physical and psychological trauma. Of course, there may be physical trauma to the victim and others. Varying degrees of psychological trauma may also result depending on how "close" an individual is to the accident or victim. Everyone is affected somehow. As the length of time after an accident increases, thoughts and emotions distort what people believe they saw and heard. Conversations with others further distort reality. After a while, the memory of everyone associated in any way with the accident will be altered in some way. With that in mind, it's important to get written statements and conduct interviews as soon as possible."[5]

An interesting side issue refers to an "internal" investigation by the employer itself.

It also notes those conducting an official OSHA accident investigation have to be careful of any "confidential" information that comes into their possession:

As stated:

"Notably, the case affirms that when an employer "has taken the important step of protecting a sensitive, detailed internal accident investigation report properly with solicitor-client privilege," it cannot be seized by Ontario's Ministry of Labour (MOL), says Jeremy Warning, a senior associate at Heenan Blaikie LLP in Toronto and a former lawyer with the MOL. "Ensuring that probing and detailed internal accident

investigations remain confidential and are not used by [oh&s] enforcers and Crown prosecutors to advance their case is a key element in an employer's accident response plan."[6]

In looking at the court recordings, the case as cited at paragraph 1 involved:

"[1] This case comes to the court by way of leave to appeal from the Ontario Court of Justice on two questions:

> *(i)   When the Crown has come into possession of a defence document that is protected by solicitor-client and litigation privilege, does the accused bear the burden of proving actual prejudice or will prejudice be presumed?*

> *(ii)   Additionally, in such circumstances, must the charges be stayed or is a lesser remedy appropriate?"*[7]

As further cited:

"[3]   On January 21, 2002, an employee of Vipond Inc., a subcontractor of Bruce Power Inc., was seriously injured in a fall while working at the nuclear power plant in Tiverton, Ontario.

[4]   On the day of the accident, Inspector Peter Martin (the "Inspector") of the Ministry of Labour (the "MOL") attended at the power plant and commenced an investigation into the accident.

[5]   Immediately after the accident, in-house counsel for Bruce Power contacted outside counsel for legal advice in anticipation that charges would be laid by the MOL under the OHSA.

[6]   Outside counsel advised that Bruce Power undertake its own investigation of the accident with the purpose of producing a report for use by counsel in providing legal advice to the company and its employees and for use in the defence of the anticipated charges under the OHSA against the company and its employees."[8]

The key facts included:

"[7]   On the day following the accident, an investigation team was created, which included both management and union employees. Ian Ritchie, a representative of the Power Workers' Union, was a member of the team. Terms of reference were produced, which expressly provided that the investigation was undertaken in contemplation of litigation and that all documents created during the investigation, including the investigation report, were to be placed in the custody of Bruce Power's legal department where their confidentiality would be maintained.

[8]   Five members of the investigative team, including Mr. Ritchie, conducted interviews of a number of people between January 22, 2002 and February 4, 2002. The people who were interviewed were expressly told, prior to the interview, that any report of the interview would remain confidential for use by legal counsel in anticipation of the charges under the OHSA. They were also advised that information obtained from the interviews would not be provided to the MOL or any other third party."[9]

Confidentiality was the key term or intention:

"[9]   A draft investigation report was prepared and was clearly marked in large, bold type, "Confidential". The draft report did not identify people by name. However, people were identified by their job classification or job description. It was circulated to team members with instructions in writing to keep the information confidential. They were also instructed to return or destroy all copies of the report in their possession."[10]

The problem for the Crown:

"[14]   On April 29, 2004, the Inspector, in the company of Crown counsel, from the MOL, responsible for prosecuting the charges, attended the home of Mr. Ritchie. During the course of that meeting, counsel for the Crown and the Inspector came into possession of a copy of the report, which Mr. Ritchie had undertaken to destroy. In the proceedings before the justice of the peace, she was unable to conclude whether Mr. Ritchie volunteered the document or whether Crown counsel and the Inspector requested it. What is clear from the findings of fact of the justice of the peace is that the Inspector was fully aware, since early 2002, that the document was subject to a claim of privilege."[11]

At the lower court, the Justice of the Peace found:

"[22]   The justice of the peace delivered her decision on the privilege issue on March 23, 2005. The justice of the peace observed that the report "does not contain within it any legal strategy or thoughts or opinions of legal counsel." She described the report as "primarily informational in its content." However, in her subsequent reasons in the second phase she also said:

The report clearly sets out items that could well be used to the disadvantage and prejudice of the defendants in these pro-ceedings and were intended to be privileged.

[23]   In her review of the evidence, the justice of the peace said:

It is clear from the evidence presented that both Mr. Martelli [in-house counsel] and Ms. Fields [outside counsel] continually stressed with the members of the Investigative Team that the report was being prepared in anticipation of litigation and was privileged, and not to be released to anyone outside of the legal department or the Investigative Team. The evidence disclosed that Mr. Martelli went so far as to attend a meeting in order to explain the meaning of the document being prepared in anticipation of litigation and the privilege that would attach to it.

[24]   The justice of the peace concluded that the report was subject to both solicitor-client and litigation privilege. She also concluded that the privilege had not been waived. As a result, she ordered that the Crown return the original report obtained from Mr. Ritchie, any copies that had been made of the report and any notes that related to the contents of the report."[12]

The Crown appealed the lower court decision:

"[35]   The Crown appealed the decision of the justice of the peace to the Ontario Court of Justice. The appeal was heard in the spring of 2007 by the Honourable Justice Julia A. Morneau. Judgment was delivered on November 13, 2007."[13]

The Appeal Court did emphasize that solicitor-client privilege is fundamental to the administration of justice in Canada:

"[42]   At the outset I should make it clear that the finding that the report is protected by solicitor-client and litigation privilege is not challenged in this court.

[43]   The Supreme Court of Canada has made it abundantly clear that solicitor-client privilege is fundamental to the administration of justice in Canada. It is no longer simply an evidentiary rule and has become a general principle of substantive law: see Maranda v. Richer, 2003 SCC 67 (CanLII), [2003] 3 S.C.R. 193.

[44]   In Canada (Privacy Commissioner) v. Blood Tribe Department of Health, 2008 SCC 44 (CanLII), [2008] 2 S.C.R. 574, at para. 9, Binnie J. said:

Solicitor-client privilege is fundamental to the proper func-tioning of our legal system. The complex of rules and procedures is such that, realistically speaking, it cannot be navigated without a lawyer's expert advice. It is said that anyone who represents himself or herself has a fool for a client, yet a lawyer's advice is only as good as the factual information the client provides. Experience shows that people who have a legal problem will often not make a clean breast of the facts to a lawyer without an assurance of confidentiality "as close to absolute as possible":

[S]olicitor-client privilege must be as close to absolute as possible to ensure public confidence and retain relevance. As such, it will only yield in certain clearly defined circumstances, and does not involve a balancing of interests on a case-by-case basis. [Citations omitted.]

[45]   In R. v. McClure, 2001 SCC 14 (CanLII), [2001] 1 S.C.R. 445, Major J. said at paras. 2 and 4:

Solicitor-client privilege describes the privilege that exists between a client and his or her lawyer. This privilege is fundamental to the justice system in Canada. The law is a complex web of interests, relationships and rules. The integrity of the administration of justice depends upon the unique role of the solicitor who provides legal advice to clients within this complex system. At the heart of this privilege lies the concept that people must be able to speak candidly with their lawyers and so enable their interests to be fully represented.

Solicitor-client privilege and the right to make full answer and defence are integral to our system of justice.

[46]   Finally, in *Lovalee, Rackel & Heintz v. Canada (Attorney General), 2002 SCC 61 (CanLII), [2002] 3 S.C.R. 209, at para. 36, Arbour J. said:*

Indeed, solicitor-client privilege must remain as close to absolute as possible if it is to retain relevance. Accordingly, this Court is compelled in my view to adopt stringent norms to ensure its protection."[14]

The questions for the Appeal Court included, "When the Crown has come into possession of a defence document that is protected by solicitor-client and litigation privilege, does the accused bear the burden of proving actual prejudice or will prejudice be presumed?"[15]

In answering this question, the Appeal Court referred to:

"[52]   The answer to this question is clearly found in the reasons for judgment of Binnie J. in Celanese Canada Inc. v. Murray Demolition Corp., 2006 SCC 36 (CanLII), [2006] 2 S.C.R. 189, at para. 3:

This Court's decision in MacDonald Estate v. Martin, 1990 CanLII 32 (SCC), [1990] 3 S.C.R. 1235, makes it clear that prejudice will be presumed to flow from an opponent's access to relevant solicitor-client confidences. The major difference between the minority and majority in that case is that while the majority considered the presumption of risk of prejudice open to rebuttal in some circumstances (pp. 1260-61), the minority would not have permitted even the opportunity of rebuttal (p. 1266).

[53]   Celanese involved the execution of an Anton Piller order that resulted in documents of the defendants, which were protected by solicitor-client privilege, falling into the hands of the lawyers for the plaintiffs. Binnie J. distinguished the case from the "moving solicitor" situation in MacDonald Estate. He discussed the kind of rebuttal evidence that would be expected from the party who obtained improper access to the privileged documents at para. 4.

The Anton Piller situation is somewhat different because the searching solicitors ought to have a record of exactly what was seized and what material, for which confidentiality is claimed, they subsequently looked at. Here again, rebuttal should be permitted, but the rebuttal evidence should require the party who obtained access to disclose to the court what has been learned and the measures taken to avoid the presumed resulting prejudice. While all solicitor confidences are not of the same order of importance, the party who obtained the wrongful access is not entitled to have the court assume in its favour that such disclosure carried no risk of prejudice to its opponent, and therefore does not justify the removal of the solicitors. For the reasons that follow, I conclude, contrary to the view taken by the Court of Appeal, with respect, that Celanese and its lawyers did have the onus to rebut the presumption of a risk of prejudice and they failed to do so. [Emphasis in original.]

[54] Celanese involved the removal of the solicitors for the plaintiffs from the case. That said, I see no difference in principle between the situations in MacDonald Estate and Celanese and the case at bar.

[55] Counsel for the Crown in this court sought to distinguish Celanese on the basis that it was a civil case in which the appellants were "attempting to utilize a civil onus to achieve a criminal result". I reject this submission. In my view, the above cases support the proposition that when the Crown comes into possession of a defence document that is protected by solicitor-client and litigation privilege, prejudice to the defence will be presumed. The presumption, however, is rebuttable."[16]

As such, was this a case that warranted a stay of proceedings against Bruce Power Inc.?

The Court of Appeal found:

"[66] I would allow the appeal and restore the stay of the proceedings on the charges against the appellants.

[67] Finally, I return to the two questions raised by this appeal. In respect of the first question, I would conclude that when the Crown has come into possession of a defence document that is protected by solicitor-client and litigation privilege, prejudice will be presumed."[17]

As such, it is paramount that the accident scene not be interfered with so that the OSHA accident investigator can do a proper job.

And, as a consequence, one must answer OHS investigators' questions as this next court case emphasizes.

The accident, as cited:

"[1] On March 17, 2004 a worker was killed in a workplace accident at a facility located north of Standard, Alberta ("the Accident"). Two occupational health and safety officers ("OHS officers") were assigned pursuant to the Occupational Health and Safety

Act, R.S.A. 2000 c. O-2 ("the OHS Act") to investigate the Accident. The OHS officers work in the department known as Workplace Health and Safety ("WHS")."[18]

The issue for this court, as stated:

"[2]   Mark Ebsworth ("the Applicant") was employed by the same employer as the deceased. He witnessed the Accident. Section 19(2) of the OHS Act provides that a witness shall on the request of an OHS officer, provide any information relating to an accident the OHS officer requests. Section 19(5) provides that any such statement is not admissible in evidence for any purpose in a trial, public inquiry under the Fatality Inquiries Act or other proceeding except to prove non-compliance with this section (providing information) or a contravention of section 41(3) (making a false statement or knowingly giving false information). The penalty for providing false information is a fine of not more than $1000 or imprisonment for a term not exceeding 6 months or both fine and imprisonment.

[3]   The Applicant was interviewed with his counsel present and gave a statement. The WHS subsequently changed its policy with respect to allowing counsel to be present during interviews. A second interview was requested of the Applicant in the absence of counsel.

[4]   The Applicant seeks a declaration that the OHS officers have no authority or jurisdiction under the OHS Act or at common law to exclude counsel from being present during an interview, a declaration that the Applicant's Charter rights have been, or will be, infringed, and an injunction enjoining the OHS officers from interviewing the Applicant in the absence of counsel.

[5]   The central issue is whether the Applicant is entitled to presence of counsel in circumstances where he is compelled to give a statement pursuant to s. 19(2) of the OHS Act ..

[28]   Although it may be desirable and perhaps even advantageous for all parties, to permit the presence of legal counsel during an interview conducted pursuant to s. 19 of the OHS Act, the issues are whether WHS has the jurisdiction in governing its procedure to exclude the presence of legal counsel and whether such exclusion in these circumstances contravenes the Charter.. "[19]

The employer [applicant] countered with:

"[21]   The Applicant submits that if the legislators had intended to provide an OHS officer with the power or authority to exclude a person from a witness interview they would have provided clear language of such intent in the OHS Act and the fact that the legislators were silent on the issue indicates that they had no such intention. The Applicant further submits that a public authority may not act outside its powers and that a statutorily appointed OHS officer is constrained to act within the scope of the authority

provided in the enabling statute. The Applicant argues that as there is no express authority under the Act for an OHS officer to exclude counsel from a witness interview, any attempt by an OHS officer to do so is ultra vires.

[22]   The Applicant further submits that the policy of prohibiting witnesses from having legal counsel present at an investigative interview is unconstitutional, as it is contrary to ss. 7 and 10 of the Canadian Charter of Rights and Freedoms ("Charter"). Further, the statutory obligation to provide information to an OHS officer breaches a witness's right against self-incrimination and right to silence, contrary to ss. 7, 11(c), and 13 of the Charter.

[23]   The Applicant also submits that the policy of refusing to provide a witness with a copy of their own written or oral statement is contrary to the Freedom of Information and Protection of Privacy Act, R.S.A. 2000, c. F-25 ("FOIPPA")."[20]

In looking at jurisprudence, the court cited:

"[31]   In Irvine v. Canada (Restrictive Trade Practices Commission) 1987 CanLII 81 (SCC), [1987] 1 S.C.R. 181 the Supreme Court held that an investigative body must have control of its own procedure, and where the legislation in question did not expressly provide a right to cross-examine witnesses and the duty of fairness did not require it, the hearing officer could refuse to permit cross-examination (para. 78). Similarly here the OHS officers have the right to control their procedures, as long as they do not conflict with the OHS Act."[21]

The employer [applicant] countered with:

"[32]   The Applicant points to legislation in other provinces which expressly provides that a person who is questioned may be accompanied by another person if they wish: Workers' Compensation Act, S.B.C. 1996, c. 492, s. 179(3)(h), Workplace Safety and Health Act, C.C.S.M. c. W120, s. 24(1)(k), Occupational Health and Safety Act, R.S.N.S. 1996, c. 7, ss. 50(6) and (7), Occupational Health and Safety Act, R.S.P.E.I., c. O-1, 7(4). The legislative provisions in Ontario give the officers discretion to determine who may attend: Occupational Health and Safety Act, R.S.O., c. 0.1, s. 54(1)(h) ["an officer may question any person who is or was in a workplace either separate and apart from another person or in the presence of any other person..."]. The Applicant argues that these illustrate that the legislatures have recognized that the power to allow or exclude attendance, if desired, must be expressly granted to an officer."[22]

The court replied:

"[33]   I disagree. If the legislation expressly stated that a person may request that someone accompany him, OHS officers could not exclude legal counsel, but that does not

mean that, where the legislation is silent, the OHS officers have no ability to set their own procedure for investigations...

[35]   Moreover, s. 25(2) of the Interpretation Act, R.S.A. 2000, c. I -8 provides that:
(2) If in an enactment power is given to a person to do or enforce the doing of any act or thing, all other powers that are necessary to enable the person to do or enforce the doing of the act or thing are deemed to be given also. "[23]

The employer [applicant] also alleged Charter violation:

"[38]   The Applicant argues that his rights under ss. 7 and 10 of the Charter have been breached, and will continue to be breached, if the Respondent is permitted to compel a statement from him in the absence of his legal counsel. It is important to note that it is the combination of the compelled statement and refusal to allow legal counsel to attend that forms the basis of the Applicant's claim.

[39]   Sections 7 and 10 of the Charter provide:

7. Everyone has the right to life, liberty and security of the person and the right not to be deprived thereof except in accordance with the principles of fundamental justice.

10. Everyone has the right on arrest or detention

a) to be informed promptly of the reasons therefor;

b) to retain and instruct counsel without delay and to be informed of that right; and

c) to have the validity of the detention determined by way of habeas corpus and to be released if the detention is not lawful.

[40]   The Applicant notes that it is important to consider context in assessing a Charter claim, citing Fitzpatrick v. The Queen, 1995 CanLII 44 (SCC), [1995] 4 S.C.R. 154, 102 C.C.C. (3d) 144 (at p. 157):

... in Wholesale Travel, supra, at p. 243 C.C.C., p. 211 D.L.R., Cory J. held that "a Charter right may have different scope and implications in a regulatory context than in a truly criminal one", and that "constitutional standards developed in the criminal context cannot be applied automatically to regulatory offences". These comments must be borne in mind in approaching the appellant's claims, for it is made in the context of a detailed regulatory regime that governs state conservation and management of the fishery. In this regulatory environment, we must be careful to avoid automatically applying rules that have been developed respecting self - incrimination in the criminal sphere. "[24]

The court rebutted with:

"[41]   In this case, the context includes the fact that the OHS Act provides no right to remain silent and no protection against self-incrimination, since the Applicant is required to provide a statement, and failure to do so is an offence that could result in imprisonment. This requirement to provide a statement is off-set by a limited use clause in s. 19(5), that any statement given in an investigation is not admissible in any proceeding except for a proceeding against the witness for failing to provide a statement or for providing a false statement, an offence under s. 41(3)...

[63]   The gathering of information in the OHS investigation is similar to the routine information gathering in the immigration situation. The Applicant's liberty interest is not in jeopardy, and the risk of future charges arising from the statement is not an imminent one. Further, his psychological integrity is not threatened; "the ordinary stresses and anxieties that a person of reasonable sensibility would suffer as a result of government action" are not sufficient (G.(J.) at para. 59).

[64]   Thus, I conclude that the Applicant's rights under s. 7 have not been engaged since there is no real or imminent deprivation of liberty. Further, even if there is an attenuated risk to his liberty interest occasioned by the possibility of imprisonment for failing to provide a statement, or for providing a false statement, it has not been infringed in a manner that is inconsistent with the principles of fundamental justice. In these circumstances the principles of fundamental justice do not require that his legal counsel be present during the interview, nor does it involve a right to silence. The statutory compulsion to provide information is also consistent with fundamental justice."[25]

As such, the pertinent conclusions, as cited:

"[69]   Having considered the submissions of the parties I find that:

1.   Although it may be desirable and perhaps even advantageous to permit the presence of legal counsel during an interview conducted pursuant to s. 19 of the OHS Act, the WHS has the jurisdiction to govern its procedure and to exclude the presence of legal counsel.

2.   The policy of prohibiting witnesses from having legal counsel present during an investigative interview pursuant to section 19 of the OHS Act is not contrary to the Charter."[26]

Footnotes

1 - 5. 702 Accident Investigation
Steven J. Geigle, MA, CET, CSHM
OSHAcademy Safety and Health Training
www.oshatrain.org

6. *Privileged Information: Hands-Off Documents*
By Dan Birch
Dec 2009
http://www.ohscanada.com/lawfile/HandsOffDocuments.aspx

7 – 17. *R. v. Bruce Power Inc., 2009 ONCA 573 (CanLII)*
Date: 2009-07-17
Docket: C49091
Parallel citations: 245 CCC (3d) 315
http://www.canlii.org/eliisa/highlight.do?text=R.+v.+Bruce+Power+Inc&language=en&s
earchTitle=Ontario&path=/en/on/onca/doc/2009/2009onca573/2009onca573.html

18 - 26. *Ebsworth v. Alberta (Human Resources and Employment), 2005 ABQB 976
(CanLII)*
Date: 2005-12-20
Docket: 0403 11491
Parallel citations: 396 AR 345; 137 CRR (2d) 49
http://www.canlii.org/eliisa/highlight.do?text=ohs+fines&language=en&searchTitle=Sear
ch+all+CanLII+Databases&path=/en/ab/abqb/doc/2005/2005abqb976/2005abqb976.html

Chapter 6 - Not adverse economic consequence

These court cases emphasize, it a court finds the costs of a fine are not considered adverse economic consequence to the employer, the fine imposed will not be adjusted.

A number of court cases exemplify that principle.

They also give the reader an idea for which type of infractions Administrative Penalties are issued.

3051939 Nova Scotia Limited (Hearthstone Inn)

In this case, as cited at paragraph 1:

"On November 01, 2010, pursuant to Section 4(1) of the Occupational Health and Safety Administrative Penalties Regulations (hereinafter referred to as the "OHS Administrative Penalties Regulations"), the Administrator issued:

- Administrative Penalty #1000127821-001 in the amount of $500.00,
- Administrative Penalty#1000127821-002 in the amount of $500.00,
- Administrative Penalty#1000127821-004 in the amount of $500.00 and
-Administrative Penalty#1000127821-010 in the amount of $500.00 to 3051939 Nova Scotia Limited, operating as Hearthstone Inn ("the Appellant")."[1]

In response, the employer [appellant] sought a reduction of the Administrative Penalty:

"On December 14, 2010, pursuant to Section 11 of the OHS Administrative Penalties Regulations, the Appellant filed an Appeal with the Occupational Health and Safety Appeal Panel ("Appeal Panel") requesting that consideration be given to reducing the fines for each Penalty to $100.00."[2]

The court noted, in determining this issue found that:

"[42]   I am satisfied that there is no evidence before me as to any efforts made by the Appellant to prevent the contravention from occurring."[3]

Concluding at paragraph 104 that the Administrative Penalty (ies) will not be reduced:

"[104]   In conclusion, the decision of the Appeal Panel on the Administrative Penalties in question is as follows:

Administrative Penalty #1000127821-001 is confirmed in the amount of $500.00.

Administrative Penalty #1000127821-002 is confirmed in the amount of $500.00.

Administrative Penalty #1000127821-004 is confirmed in the amount of $500.00.

Administrative Penalty #1000127821-010 is confirmed in the amount of $500.00."[4]

Nima Vani Enterprises

In this case, as cited at paragraphs 1 and 3:

"[1]   On October 14, 2010, pursuant to Section 4(1) of the Occupational Health and Safety Administrative Penalties Regulations (hereinafter referred to as the "OHS Administrative Penalties Regulations"), the Administrator issued:

- Administrative Penalty #1000128243-003 in the amount of $500.00,
- Penalty #1000128243-005 in the amount of $400.00 and
- Penalty #1000128243-007 in the amount of $500.00 to Nima Vani Enterprises ("the Appellant")."[5]

The infractions included:

"Order #1000128243-003 re: Occupational Health and Safety First Aid Regulations, 5-3-a First-aid Certificates: lack of trained first aiders as per the first-aid regulations thus resulting in an order and an administrative penalty.

Order #1000128243-005 re: Occupational Safety General Regulations, 25-1 Fire Protection and Escape: lack of certified extinguishers on site thus resulting in an order and an administrative penalty.

Order #1000128243-007 re: Violence in the Workplace Regulations, 5-1 Violence Risk assessment: lack of a Violence risk assessment thus resulting in an order and an administrative penalty."[6]

Likewise, in response, the employer [appellant] sought that the Administrative Penalties be waived:

"On November 1, 2010 pursuant to Section 11 of the OHS Administrative Penalties Regulations, the Appellant filed an Appeal with the Occupational Health and Safety Appeal Panel ("Appeal Panel") requesting the penalties to be waived."[7]

Again the court found that:

"[17]   I am satisfied that the Appellant made little or no effort to prevent the violation from occurring."[8]

Likewise, the court concluding at paragraph 79 that the Administrative Penalties will not be waived:

"[79]   In conclusion, the decision of the Appeal Panel on the Administrative Penalties in question are as follows:

   Administrative Penalty #1000128243-003 is confirmed in the amount of $500.00.

   Administrative Penalty #1000128243-005 is confirmed in the amount of $400.00.

   Administrative Penalty #1000128243-007 is confirmed in the amount of $500.00."[9]

Gary Belliveau Construction and Excavation Ltd

In this case, as cited at paragraphs 1:

"[1]   On October 21, 2010, pursuant to Section 4(1) of the Occupational Health and Safety Administrative Penalties Regulations (hereinafter referred to as the "OHS Administrative Penalties Regulations"), the Administrator issued Administrative Penalty #1012410556-002 in the amount of $1,000.00, Penalty #1012410556-004 in the amount of $500.00 and Penalty #1012410556-006 in the amount of $400.00 to Gary Belliveau Construction and Excavation Ltd. ("the Appellant")."[10]

Likewise, in response, the employer [appellant] sought that the Administrative Penalties be waived:

"On October 27, 2010 pursuant to Section 11 of the OHS Administrative Penalties Regulations, the Appellant filed an Appeal with the Occupational Health and Safety Appeal Panel ("Appeal Panel") requesting the penalties be waived."[11]

More specifically at paragraph 3 it was cited:

"[3]   On August 10, 2010 an OHS inspector conducted an inspection at 455 Little Brook Road, Little Brookk, NS. The workplace is a construction project that involves a renovation to a former hardware store by a new owner. Employees were in the process of re-shingling the north side of the roof. The building is 50' long and 40' wide. The edge of the roof is approximately 20' high and the roof has a 4/12 pitch. An inspection was conducted at the workplace after observing employees working on the roof without having a fully decked scaffold or roof brackets and planks at the edge of the roof. There were 7 orders issued and 3 of those orders warranted Administrative Fines.

Order #1012410556-002 re: Fall Protection and Scaffolding Regulations, 7-1 Fall Protection Required: employees were working 3 meters or more above a safe surface and were not adequately protected from falling by wearing an adequate fall arrest system or working within the confines of an adequately constructed guardrail thus resulting in an order and an administrative penalty.

In their Appeal, the Appellant submits that "we find it is an outrageously high amount for a first offence. We have upgraded the required safety equipment and feel that these penalties are excessively high for a first offence considering our past safety record". As such, the Appellant requests that the administrative penalty in question be removed.

Order #1000128243-004 re: Fall Protection and Scaffolding Regulations, 27 Metal Scaffolds: metal scaffolds were improperly erected as required by the regulations thus resulting in an order and an administrative penalty.

In their Appeal, the Appellant submits that "in our opinion staging was erected using proper legs and a sound foundation. Staging was stable". As such, the Appellant requests that the administrative penalty in question be removed.

Order #1000128243-006 re: Occupational Safety General Regulations, 11 Hazard to Head: employees were not wearing head protection as required by the regulations thus resulting in an order and an administrative penalty.

In their Appeal, the Appellant submits that "Hard Hats...this is excessive for a first offence. Our understanding that a person working above on the staging was not required to wear head protection". As such, the Appellant requests that the administrative penalty in question be removed."[12]

The court also noted:

"[9]   In his submission, the Director submits that" in issuing the compliance order, the OHS Officer, in consideration of the circumstances of the matter, noted that here was potential for injury or risk of immediate injury"."[13]

As such, the court indicated a greater Administrative Penalty was in order:

"[11]   I have reviewed the records considered by the Administrator as well as the submissions and evidence from the Appellant and Director and find that the base amount of $1,000.00 is appropriate in this case."[14]

Likewise, the court concluding at paragraph 79 that the Administrative Penalties will not be waived:

"[79]   In conclusion, the decision of the Appeal Panel on the Administrative Penalties in question are as follows:

Administrative Penalty #1012410556-002 is confirmed in the amount of $1,000.00.

Administrative Penalty #1012410556-004 is confirmed in the amount of $500.00.

Administrative Penalty #1012410556-006 is confirmed in the amount of $400.00."[15]

Jim Kirk Carpentry Services Limited

In this case, as cited at paragraphs 1:

"[1]   On October 18 and 20, 2010, pursuant to Section 4(1) of the Occupational Health and Safety Administrative Penalties Regulations (hereinafter referred to as the "OHS Administrative Penalties Regulations"), the Administrator issued:

- Administrative Penalty #1013810543-002 in the amount of $400.00,

-penalty #1013810543-003 in the amount of $1000.00 and

-penalty #1013810543-005 in the amount of $400.00 to Jim Kirk Carpentry Services Limited ("the Appellant")."[16]

Specifically, at paragraph 3:

"[3]   On August 5, 2010 this Officer visited Jim Kirk Carpentry Services Limited, client at the RK MacDonald Nursing Home. The Establishment is building an addition to the home and have employed APM construction as the general contractor. APM Construction has in turn hired the above noted contractor to construct, coordinate sub trades and supervise site activities. As a result of this visit 3 Warnings and 5 Orders were issued, as follows:

Warning (1) An employer shall maintain and service the fire protection equipment required in subsection (1) in accordance with the manufacturer's specifications. Warning (2) The employer shall ensure the step ladder with bent support braces is removed from service until repaired or replaced; and ensure the half step ladder is repaired or replaced, properly maintained, secured when in use, and extensions at least 3 rungs above the safe surface that is being accessed. Warning (3) The employer shall ensure power operated hand grinder are maintained with the guards in place and that the grinding discs are replaced as per the manufacturers specifications.

Order #1013810543-001 The wall brackets must be taken down and isolated to prevent further use, at this workplace or any other employer workplace, workplace, until there is compliance with Order(s) 1013810543-002 and Stop Work #1013810543-001 is withdrawn or cancelled by an officer, must be complied with by August 5, 2010.

Order #1013810543-002 The employer shall ensure the wall bracket scaffolds are engineered designed, operated in accordance with written procedures, and, used and maintained in accordance with the professional engineers instructions, as required by the regulations. Must be complied with by August 5, 2010, resulted in Administrative Penalty which was appealed by the Appellant.

Order #1013810543-003 The employer shall ensure the end frame scaffolds are erected, used, maintained and dismantled in accordance with the manufacturers specifications, as per this regulation, Issued Under the Occupational Health and Safety Act. Must be complied with by August 12, 2010, resulted in Administrative Penalty, was appealed by the Appellant.

Order #1013810543-004 The employer shall ensure the rolling scaffold is erected with horizontal cross brace with locking mechanisms, as required by the regulation, must be complied with by August 12, 2010.

Order #1013810543-005 The employer shall ensure the two excavations on the College Street side of the building are adequately fenced, guarded or barricaded as required by the regulation, must be complied with by August 13, 2010. This contravention occurred on August 9, 2010, resulted in Administrative Penalty which was appealed by the Appellant."[17]

On appeal, the company stated:

"[4]   In their appeal letter the Appellant submits that "We do agree things were not quite the way they should have been, but when items were brought to our attention by thr Dept. of Labour Office, we complied immediately by removing the items from the site that she requested and making corrective measures to all the other items." In regulation to Order # 1013810543-005, the Appellant further submits that "My company (JKCS) was not performing the trenching job @ the RK MacDonald site... The penalty, if applicable, should meted to the construction company paid to do this job."[18]

In deciding, the court mentioned:

"[17]   I am satisfied that the Appellant made some efforts to prevent the violation from occurring."[19]

Likewise, the court concluding at paragraph 79 that the Administrative Penalties will not be waived:

"[79]   In conclusion, the decision of the Board on the Administrative Penalties in question is as follows:

Administrative Penalty #1013810543-002 is confirmed in the amount of $400.00.

Administrative Penalty #1013810543-003 is confirmed in the amount of $1000.00.

Administrative Penalty #1013810543-005 is confirmed in the amount of $400.00."[20]

Footnotes

1 - 4. *3051939 Nova Scotia Limited (Hearthstone Inn) (Re), 2011 NSOHSAP 136 (CanLII)*
Date: 2011-07-22
Docket: OHS-0276
http://www.canlii.org/eliisa/highlight.do?text=ohs+fines&language=en&searchTitle=Search+all+CanLII+Databases&path=/en/ns/nsohsap/doc/2011/2011nsohsap136/2011nsohsap136.html

5 - 9. *Nima Vani Enterprises (Re), 2011 NSOHSAP 93 (CanLII)*
Date: 2011-05-02
Docket: OHS-0240
http://www.canlii.org/eliisa/highlight.do?text=ohs+fines&language=en&searchTitle=Search+all+CanLII+Databases&path=/en/ns/nsohsap/doc/2011/2011nsohsap93/2011nsohsap93.html

10 - 15. *Gary Belliveau Construction and Excavation Ltd (Re), 2011 NSOHSAP 92 (CanLII)*
Date: 2011-05-02
Docket: OHS-0241
http://www.canlii.org/eliisa/highlight.do?text=ohs+fines&language=en&searchTitle=Search+all+CanLII+Databases&path=/en/ns/nsohsap/doc/2011/2011nsohsap92/2011nsohsap92.html

16 - 20. *Jim Kirk Carpentry Services Limited (Re), 2012 NSLB 38 (CanLII)*
Date: 2012-01-31
Docket: OHS-0249
http://www.canlii.org/eliisa/highlight.do?text=ohs+fines&language=en&searchTitle=Search+all+CanLII+Databases&path=/en/ns/nslb/doc/2012/2012nslb38/2012nslb38.html

Chapter 7 - Reporting Fatalities and Hospitalizations

There is a requirement to report accidents.

As cited under Section 1904.39:

"(a) Basic requirement. Within eight (8) hours after the death of any employee from a work-related incident or the in-patient hospitalization of three or more employees as a result of a work-related incident, you must orally report the fatality/multiple hospitalization by telephone or in person to the Area Office of the Occupational Safety and Health Administration (OSHA), U.S. Department of Labor, that is nearest to the site of the incident. You may also use the OSHA toll-free central telephone number, 1-800-321-OSHA (1-800-321-6742).

(b) Implementation—(1) If the Area Office is closed, may I report the incident by leaving a message on OSHA's answering machine, faxing the area office, or sending an e-mail? No, if you can't talk to a person at the Area Office, you must report the fatality or multiple hospitalization incident using the 800 number.

(2) What information do I need to give to OSHA about the incident? You must give OSHA the following information for each fatality or multiple hospitalization incident:

(i) The establishment name;

(ii) The location of the incident;

(iii) The time of the incident;

(iv) The number of fatalities or hospitalized employees;

(v) The names of any injured employees;

(vi) Your contact person and his or her phone number; and

(vii) A brief description of the incident."[1]

This also includes:

"(5) Do I have to report a fatality caused by a heart attack at work? Yes, your local OSHA Area Office director will decide whether to investigate the incident, depending on the circumstances of the heart attack."[2]

And:

"(7) What if I don't learn about an incident right away? If you do not learn of a reportable incident at the time it occurs and the incident would otherwise be reportable under paragraphs (a) and (b) of this section, you must make the report within eight (8) hours of the time the incident is reported to you or to any of your agent(s) or employee(s)."[3]

In Canada, reporting an accident varies between provinces.

But, in general, as cited:

"The rules for reporting injuries are pretty standard across the country, but the penalties for non-compliance vary wildly."[4]

"All the boards require prompt accident reporting -- usually within three to five days. And all the boards have penalties for false reporting or failing to report accidents."[5]

"Ontario plays hardball, with fines that can reach $100,000, while most other jurisdictions have fines ranging up to just $5,000, and one -- New Brunswick -- assesses a maximum penalty of just $50."[6]

"Many of these jurisdictions rely on the fraud provisions of the Criminal Code of Canada to penalize employers who deliberately try to suppress claims or manipulate claims costs. However, few employers get convicted via this route."[7]

British Columbia, Canada

In British Columbia, Canada for example:

"Under Bill 14, which became law on October 1, 1999, the WCB can prosecute offenders through the provincial court system when a serious offence (such as false reporting) is involved."[8]

"Bill 14 allows the courts to impose penalties that can include fines of up to $500,000, imprisonment for a term of up to six months, or both, Pinto points out. For repeat offenders, these penalties can double."[9]

An example case under Bill 14 is cited here:

"[1]   On June 12, 2006, a blaster was killed in an accident while engaged in road construction. On the morning of the accident, the blaster forgot to bring his blasting equipment to the work site from the nearby town in which they were staying. He attempted to set off the blast using make-shift materials available at the construction site (including used firing line which had been discarded). There were several unsuccessful attempts to set off the blast. The co-workers connected the firing line to a truck battery and set about repairing breaks in the line and checking it for continuity using a light

bulb. The blast occurred unexpectedly while the blaster was at the blast site. Toxicology results indicated the blaster's judgment may have been impaired due to use of cocaine.

[2]   By decision dated August 3, 2007, an occupational safety officer (OSO) of the Workers' Compensation Board, operating as WorkSafeBC (Board or WCB), imposed an administrative penalty of $200,000.00 under section 196 of the Workers Compensation Act (Act), and a claim costs levy of $16,100.29, under section 73(1) of the Act. (For brevity, in this decision the term "penalty" is used to mean "administrative penalty.") [10]

As further cited:

"[7]   The employer does not dispute that the events on June 12, 2006, which resulted in the death of the blaster, involved violations of the Act and the Occupational Health and Safety Regulation (Regulation) for which a penalty is warranted ... Related questions in this appeal include:

(a)   did the worker's death on June 12, 2006 result from the employer committing a high risk violation wilfully or with reckless disregard?

(b)   did the employer obstruct the OSO's investigation?

(c)   did the OSO issue a verbal order to the employer on June 13, 2006, not to conduct further blasting until it had developed and implemented enhanced written procedures for blasting?

(d)   did the employer conduct two further blasts on June 17 and 21, 2006, before developing and implementing enhanced written procedures for blasting?

(e)   did the employer proceed with further blasting in October and November 2006, after its replacement blaster's certificate expired?

(f)   should a penalty be imposed under the table for a Category A penalty, or should it be a discretionary penalty?

(g)   if a claim costs levy is imposed, what significance attaches to the fact Ms. X has an appeal before WCAT seeking benefits under section 17 of the Act?" [11]

As further cited, during the oral hearing, evidence by the OSO included:

"[64]   The OSO gave evidence under oath. He had worked as the blasting coordinator for the Board, and had been a certified blaster for 33 years. He summarized the violations of Part 21 of the Regulation concerning Blasting Operations which he found at the time of his inspection following the accident (with reference to the material

set out in Part B of his Recommendation for Administrative Penalty, under the heading "Officer's Decision").

[65]   *These included:*

•   *The firm's inability to produce complete blasting logs for this project.*

•   *There was evidence of unrecorded blasts (section 21.4 of the Regulation).*

•   *The firm carried on blasting in October and November 2006 without a valid blasting certificate (section 21.5). The replacement blaster advised in June 2006, that his certificate would expire in October.*

•   *The OSO observed an active burn pile near the explosives magazine, which was an extremely hazardous situation (section 21.19). Explosives came in cardboard boxes which were typically recycled or burned after use (not beside the magazine).*

•   *There was no proper inventory of materials coming in or out of the explosives magazine (section 21.36).*

•   *The firm was subject to a legal requirement to use the explosive material in the manner recommended by the manufacturer. By using a vehicle battery rather than an appropriate blasting machine, the employer was in contravention of the manufacturer's recommendations for use (section 21.36).*

[66]   *The OSO stated the most obvious violation was not having the proper equipment to do the blast. The use of a battery posed a high risk of accidental detonation, as well as sending an uncontrolled amount of current to the line (section 21.13, 21.36, 4.3(1)(b)). If it failed to detonate the charge, then the blaster would have to investigate why there had been a misfire. In some cases, the cap may have started burning but the amount of current was insufficient to fire it. He said the firm was mishandling the misfires (section 21.73). When current is put into a line, a minimum ten minute wait was required after any failure to fire so the blaster could assess the situation. The blaster attempted to fire the blast on a number of occasions, in a repetitive fashion. The blaster failed to use a blasting machine which provided a controlled amount of current. The firm did not have appropriate testing equipment to check the amount of current in the line (section 21.63). The circuit was not tested and no records were kept. The workers on site had no reasonable method to check the line.*

[67]   *The OSO stated that there was a lack of supervision of the entire operation. The blaster was permitted to carry on with unsafe work practices. The foreman was involved in work activities which contributed to the accident, while the blaster was not present. The OSO stated the blast should not have been allowed to proceed in this fashion. It was obvious the foreman knew they did not have the proper blasting equipment or firing line on site.*

[68]   The OSO provided his reasons for issuing an order regarding obstruction by the employer. He said that following the accident, the workers left the site and went home. The OSO requested that the firm make the workers available the following morning, June 13, 2006, for interviews. The firm initially agreed, but the following day the firm advised the OSO that the workers would not be available to be interviewed as they were seeking legal counsel.

[69]   The OSO stated that he also encountered resistance when he attempted to collect documentation on June 13, 2006. QA declined to provide documents to the OSO. The OSO decided to wait at the office, where P2 and a worker were present. His understanding was that they were awaiting word from P1 as to whether P1 would permit the release of documents that day. The OSO stayed in the site office until 3:00 or 3:30 p.m. but P1 did not arrive. The firm's decision not to release documents to him was not changed at that time. The OSO received the documents a few days later. The OSO stated it was very unusual for an employer to refuse to produce documents. Before leaving, he directed P2, by means of a verbal order, that there would be no more blasting on that site until such time as effective appropriate procedures for blasting activities were developed and implemented for the site. The OSO stated that he informed P2 that he would follow up on this verbal order with a written order. When the written procedures were developed and approved, he would provide the firm with a written release.

[70]   With reference to the June 21, 2006 inspection report (2006128680035), the OSO confirmed this order represented the written confirmation of his verbal order. He received the written procedures on June 28, 2006 (after attending the site to assist the employer in developing these procedures), and provided the firm with a release to conduct further blasting.

[71]   The OSO confirmed he had learned that the firm had conducted a blast during the period following his verbal stop blasting order. QA advised him in an interview on June 26, 2006 that the firm had set off a blast on the Saturday following the accident. QA confirmed he was present when the OSO gave the verbal stop blasting order to P2 on June 13, 2006."[12]

As a consequence, the court ruled:

"*[229]   ... We increase the discretionary penalty to $200,000.00, in connection with the death of the blaster on June 12, 2006 and the associated breaches of the Act and Regulation by the employer. In reaching this conclusion, we found:*

(a)   the worker's death on June 12, 2006 resulted from the employer committing a high risk violation wilfully or with reckless disregard;

(b)   the OSO issued a verbal order to the employer on June 13, 2006, not to conduct further blasting until it had developed and implemented enhanced written procedures for blasting;

(c)   the employer conducted two further blasts on June 17 and 21, 2006, before developing and implementing enhanced written procedures for blasting;

(d)   the employer proceeded with further blasting in October and November 2006, after its replacement blaster's certificate expired;

(e)   a discretionary penalty was appropriate, rather than using the table for a Category A penalty;

(f)   in levying a discretionary penalty, regard may be had to a range of factors including the size of the employer and any contribution by other parties. In exercising this discretion, no one factor need be determinative. In this case, we found that deterrence, and motivating future compliance, were paramount considerations;

(g)   even if the employer briefly obstructed the OSO's investigation while obtaining legal advice, this did not affect our consideration of the quantum of the penalty in this case; and,

(h)   a claim costs levy was properly imposed, in connection with the current costs of the claim, under section 73(1) of the Act. In the event of any increased claim costs as a result of the current appeal to WCAT by Ms. X concerning section 17 of the Act, the Board may consider as a new issue in implementing the WCAT decision whether an additional charge to the employer should be made of any such further claim costs up to the statutory maximum."[13]

Manitoba, Canada

In Manitoba, Canada it is cited:

"If a worker loses consciousness, misses work, requires medical attention or intends to seek medical attention, his or her employer must report to the WCB within five working days, says a WCB spokesperson."[14]

"If employers are late in sending in injury claims, they will be responsible for paying an administrative fee of $150. If they are chronically late, however, they can be forced to pay $5,000, spend three months in jail, or both, if found guilty under the compensation act for false reporting."[15]

An example Manitoba case is cited here:

At paragraph 5, it is noted "the applicable provisions of the Canada Labour Code, R.S.C. 1985, Chapter L2 are the following:

Duties of Employers - General duty of employer

124. Every employer shall ensure that the safety and health at work of every person employed by the employer is protected.

Specific duties of employer

125. Without restricting the generality of section 124, every employer shall, in respect of every work place controlled by the employer,

> *(b)   install guards, guardrails, barricades and fences in accordance with prescribed standards;*

> *(c)   investigate, record and report in the manner and to the authorities as prescribed all accidents, occupational diseases and other hazardous occurrences known to the employer;...*

> *(t)   ensure that the machinery, equipment and tools used by the employees in the course of their employment meet prescribed safety standards and are safe under all conditions of their intended use."*[16]

The case, as cited, at paragraphs 1 and 2 involved:

"[1]   Glen Zommer, on the 15th day of September, 2000, sustained a serious injury to his left hand while operating a DCW7000 welding machine in the course of his employment as a welder by Canadian National Railway Company in the City of Winnipeg, in Manitoba ("C.N.R.").

[2]   The investigation into this accident led to the charges against C.N.R. under the provisions of the Canada Labour Code and Canada Occupational Safety and Health Regulations."[17]

The issue before the court was:

"[7]   The sole issue in this case is due diligence and reasonable care.

[8]   The information from the exhibits and testimony of the witnesses, all of whom I find credible, is accepted as fact.

[9]   Glenn Zommer was a properly trained operator of the two plus million dollar DCW7000 welding machine utilized. His job was to weld the rail pieces together. He performed this job with this machine for the past five years.

[10]   On the 15th of September, 2000, his working shift was 15:30 to 23:30 hours. The accident occurred between 20:30 – 20:45 hours on or about the third weld after a rest break on a routine welding job.

[11]   He was watching a rail on this machine passing through in front of him. He saw a yellow chalk mark on it but saw no defect (see Exhibits 7 and 8). This mark alerted Zommer to a possible flaw.

[12]   Zommer acknowledged that if he saw the defect he must move the rail to the west of the welder to be cut out by the saw.

[13]   In this instance, he inserted his left hand into the exposed, unprotected, unobstructed, unlit and dark, tunnel-like opening for a distance of about 30 inches to feel for any flaw on that portion of the rail then beyond his visual view.

[14]   Simultaneously, with his right hand on the clamp activity button on the control panel, he caused the clamp to drop and crush his fingertips, resulting in a serious injury. This appeared to be a deliberate act and not an act of mere inadvertence.

[15]   As Zommer himself put it:

I stuck my hand to feel the flaw. The rail squashed my fingers. The clamps came down on top of the rail.

He acknowledged that he should not have inserted his hand there.

[16]   Zommer misjudged the exact location of this clamp in relation to that rail piece. The tunnel was dark and probably dark enough to obscure visually the exact location of the clamps.

[17]   Supervisor Richardson testified that after the accident he put his head into the tunnel to see the exact location of the clamps and was surprised to learn how close it was to the opening. It appears clear that Zommer also did not know how close the clamp was to the opening on this routine operation."[18]

At issue:

"[35]   The accident occurred on the Friday evening of the 15th of September, 2000. Section 15.5 of the Regulations requires the employer to report the accident to a Safety Officer as soon as possible but not later than 24 hours. It was not reported as required until Monday the 18th of September at 11:30 a.m.

[36]   The machine was cleaned on Saturday morning of the 16th of September as a normal operation. It was internally checked on Monday morning and after internally

finding that it was fully operational it was placed in full operation well before the reporting to and the arrival of the Safety Inspector on the 18th of September, 2000. Section 127 of the Labour Code prohibits the removal, interference with or disturbing anything related to the incident unless authorized to do so by a Safety Officer."[19]

In terms of due diligence, it is cited at paragraph 57:

"[57]   In my view, it is clear that regardless whether under the circumstances of, firstly, exposed moving parts or, secondly, under circumstances of processing, transporting or handling materials that constitute a hazard to an employee, the prescribed machine guard must prevent contact between the employee and the part of the machine or prevent access to the area of hazard during the operation of the machine."[20]

The court also noted:

"[97]   There is no evidence that the Labour Code and Regulations were considered by anyone on behalf of C.N.R. either when designating the specifications of the welder before Chematron manufactured it or at any time following the delivery of the welding machine to C.N.R. and during its operation. The welding machine was designed according to the specifications of C.N.R.

[98]   There is no evidence that Chematron was ever apprised of the relevant provisions of the Labour Code and Regulations.

[99]   There is no evidence that the safety inspector ever inspected singularly or regularly the operation of the welder or approved the design as compliant to the Code and Regulations.

[100]   There is no evidence that the proximity of the clamp area to the operator was ever brought to the attention of any safety inspector or operator including Zommer. There were no warning labels affixed in the vicinity of the tunnel opening leading to the clamp area advising of the exact location of the clamps and continually reminding the operator of risk in inserting a hand there during engagement of the clamps.

[101]   There is no evidence that C.N.R. ever considered installation of a control switch at the opening of the tunnel that would automatically turn off the machine and raise the clamps upon intrusion to the tunnel of anything including a hand of the operator."[21]

And:

"[103]   Negligence of an employee does not exempt C.N.R. as employer from responsibility or any statutory duty, under section 126(2) of the Canada Labour Code."[22]

With the court ruling at paragraph 127:

"[127]   Finally, as to Counts 3 and 4, upon consideration of all the evidence, the submissions by both learned counsel, the reasons and case law as discussed in the foregoing paragraphs, I find, firstly, that the prosecution proved the commission of each of them by the accused, beyond a reasonable doubt, and, secondly, that the accused failed to establish, on a balance of probabilities, due diligence and reasonable care.

The accused is, therefore, convicted of Counts 3 and 4."[23]

Those being:

"Count 3 - On or about the 15th day of September 2000, at or near the City of Winnipeg in the Province of Manitoba, the Canadian National Railway Company/Compagnie des chemins de fer nationaux du Canada, an employer within the meaning of Part II of the Canada Labour Code, did unlawfully fail to ensure that a DCW7000 welding machine, machinery used by one of its employees, Glenn Zommer, in the course of his employment was equipped with a machine guard in accordance with prescribed standards, the direct result of which was a serious injury to the employee, Glenn Zommer, contrary to paragraph 13.13(1)(b) of the Canada Occupational Safety and Health Regulations and paragraph 125(t) of the Canada Labour Code, thereby committing an offence under subsection 148(4) of the Canada Labour Code.

Count 4 - On or about the 1tth day of September 2000, at or near the City of Winnipeg in the Province of Manitoba, the Canadian National Railway Company/Compagnie des chemins de fer nationaux du Canada, an employer within the meaning of Part II of the Canada Labour Code, did unlawfully fail to ensure that a DCW7000 welding machine, machinery used by one of its employees, Glenn Zommer, in the course of his employment was equipped with a machine guard in accordance with prescribed standards, contrary to paragraph 13.13(1)(b) of the Canada Occupational Safety and Health Regulations and paragraph 125(t) of the Canada Labour Code, thereby committing an offence under subsection 148(1) of the Canada Labour Code."[24]

Ontario, Canada

In Ontario, Canada it is cited:

As cited, "the Workplace Safety and Insurance Board (WSIB) states that all injuries that require health care or result in the worker not being able to earn full wages must be reported by the employer within three days of learning of the accident, says Ted Bilger, a spokesperson from the WSIB's Special Investigations Branch (SIB)."[25]

"Ontario is clearly the most active enforcer when it comes to penalizing employers who don't report on time and/or knowingly file false or misleading claims to the WSIB. Fines and sentences levied for convictions of offences under the Workplace Safety and Insurance Act (WSIA) are ultimately decided by the court system with only the maximum sentences being specified within the act. These penalties can range up to

$25,000 for an individual and $100,000 for a corporation, although the actual fines for simple late reporting are much lower."[26]

An example case is cited here, specifically in paragraphs 1 and 2:

"1. North American Food Produce Buyers Ltd. charged and convicted for being an employer that failed to immediately notify the Ministry of Labour about its worker being critically injured in a workplace accident as required under s. 51(1) of O.H.S.A., R.S.O. 1990, c. O.1.

2. North American Food Produce Buyers Ltd. charged and convicted for being an employer who failed to provide information, instruction or supervision to its worker on the proper and safe operation of a powered pallet truck contrary to s. 25(2)(a) of O.H.S.A., R.S.O. 1990, c. O.1."[27]

And the relevant O.H.S.A. legislation includes:

"[25]   North American Produce was convicted for committing two offences under the O.H.S.A. First, it was convicted for failing to immediately report a workplace accident where a worker had been critically injured to the Ministry of Labour as required under s. 51(1) of the O.H.S.A. and secondly, it was convicted for failing to provide information, instruction and supervision to a worker about operating a powered pallet truck properly and safely to protect the health and safety of that worker, contrary to s. 25(2)(a) of the O.H.S.A.:

Notice of death or injury

51(1) Where a person is killed or critically injured from any cause at a workplace, the constructor, if any, and the employer shall notify an inspector, and the committee, health and safety representative and trade union, if any, immediately of the occurrence by telephone, telegram or other direct means and the employer shall, within forty-eight hours after the occurrence, send to a Director a written report of the circumstances of the occurrence containing such information and particulars as the regulations prescribe.

1(1)   In this Act, "inspector" means an inspector appointed for the purposes of this Act and includes a Director ... "Director" means an inspector under this Act who is appointed as a Director for the purposes of this Act;

Idem

25(2)   Without limiting the strict duty imposed by subsection (1), an employer shall,

> *(a)   provide information, instruction and supervision to a worker to protect the health or safety of the worker"[28]*

And:

"[26]   Under the O.H.S.A., a corporation convicted of an offence is liable to the penalty prescribed in s. 66(2) which provides for a fine up to a maximum of $500,000:

66(2)   If a corporation is convicted of an offence under subsection (1), the maximum fine that may be imposed upon the corporation is $500,000 and not as provided therein."[29]

With:

"On July 15, 2003, North American Produce entered guilty pleas to the two O.H.S.A. offences. As such, convictions were entered against North American Produce for failing to immediately report a workplace injury to the Ministry of Labour as required under s. 51(1) and for failing to provide information, instruction and supervision to a worker to protect the health and safety of that worker, contrary to s. 25(2)(a). In the circumstances for the first offence, although North American Produce did promptly call the police and the Workers Safety Insurance Board about the accident, it however failed as an employer to immediately inform the Ministry of Labour about the workplace accident in which one its employees was critically injured, as it was obligated to. For the second offence, North American Produce had failed as an employer to provide any training or instruction to the deceased employee about the proper and safe operation of a powered pallet truck."[30]

The circumstances:

"These are my reasons in the sentencing of North American Produce Buyers Ltd. ("North American Produce"), a corporation that has been convicted of committing two offences under the Occupational Health and Safety Act, R.S.O. 1990, c. O.1 ("O.H.S.A."). Charges were laid after a workplace accident occurred on July 23, 2001, at Toronto's Ontario Food Terminal where John Alfred Jones, an employee of North American Produce, received a crushing leg injury while operating a powered pallet truck (or power walker) in a public area. John Jones, unfortunately, died in hospital four days later from a pulmonary embolism. The autopsy that was subsequently performed on the deceased employee revealed a blot clot had obstructed blood vessels in the lungs, which then caused the employee's asphyxiation and death. However, this post-mortem examination was unable to verify that the blood clot had originated from the injured leg, which raises the question of whether Jones' death should indeed be attributed to the workplace accident."[31]

However:

"North American Produce disagrees with the Ministry of Labour's argument that this is a fatality case. In that regard, North American Produce contends that the pulmonary embolism that caused Jones' death cannot be conclusively linked to the leg injury suffered in the workplace accident and therefore, it should not be held penally liable for that unfortunate consequence. Furthermore, North American Produce suggests that

questionable medical care was the likely cause of Jones' unfortunate demise so that any prohibited act or failure to act prescribed under the O.H.S.A. that had been committed by North American Produce would not have been the cause of Jones' death."[32]

As cited at paragraph 24, the issues were:

"[24]   The following issues arise in this sentencing hearing:

(a i)   Should all harm that actually results from the workplace accident that injured the worker be attributed to North American Produce, for sentencing purposes, or should there be a limit on the consequences that can be fairly taken into account?

(a ii)   For determining the appropriate penalty or fit sentence, should North American Produce be penally liable for the death of its worker or only for the crushing leg injury that the worker suffered at the time of the accident?

(b)   Should this court for the purposes of sentencing for a regulatory offence adopt the legal causation test in Smithers v. The Queen to determine whether North American Produce should be penally liable or culpable for its employee's death or should a different causation test or analysis be used [Smithers v. The Queen, 1977 CanLII 7 (SCC), [1978] 1 S.C.R. 506 (S.C.C.)?

(d)   Is there a causal connection between North American's prohibited act or failure to train or inform its employee on the proper and safe operation of a powered pallet truck and the employee's death?

(e)   Has there been an intervening and independent act or event that could have been the cause of the worker's death?"[33]

With a disposition of:

"[74] (a) Fail to immediately notify the Ministry of Labour about the workplace accident under s. 51(1) of the O.H.S.A. - After having considered the various pertinent factors applicable to the circumstances of failing to immediately notify the Ministry of Labour of a workplace accident, in which a worker was critically injured, contrary to s. 51(1) of the Occupational Health and Safety Act, the fit or proper sentence to be imposed on North American Produce Buyers Ltd. is a fine of $12,000, exclusive of the victim fine surcharge, payable in 24 equal monthly installments of $500 on the first day of each month beginning on June 1, 2006.

[75] (b)   Fail to inform or train the employee about the proper and safe operation of the powered pallet truck under s. 25(2)(a) of the O.H.S.A. - As for the offence where North American Produce Buyers Ltd. failed to train or inform a worker about the proper and safe operation of a powered pallet truck for his health and protection contrary to s. 25(2)(a) of the Occupational Health and Safety Act, in which a worker was critically

injured, after considering the pertinent factors in relation to the circumstances of this offence, I have determined that the fit or proper sentence is the imposition of a fine of $60,000, exclusive of the victim fine surcharge, payable in 24 equal monthly installments of $2,500 on the first day of each month beginning on June 1, 2006. "[34]

The importance of workplace safety can be gleaned from the stats kept by the American Occupational Safety & Health Administration.[35]

As cited:

"Date of Incident Company and Location Preliminary Description of Incident

- *12/04/2011 Durhamtown Plantation Sportsman Resort, Union Point, GA 30669 Worker operating a bobcat at a recreational resort died when a tree limb pierced a main vein/artery.*

- *02/27/2012 Border Bin Erection LLC, Kerkhoven, MN 56252 Worker was struck by grain-bin jack.*

- *02/28/2012 Allied Waste Services of North America LLC, Bensenville, IL 60105 Worker loading a dumpster on a truck at a waste services facility was found pinned between the truck and rail system.*

- *03/02/2012 Koswire Inc., Flowery Branch, GA 30542 Worker operating a metal wiring machine was killed when he reached into the machine and was pulled in.*

- *03/02/2012 Frontier Drilling LLC, Palermo, ND 58769 Worker performing piping work died from injuries sustained when his life line broke, causing him to fall 75 feet.*

- *03/02/2012 San Saba Pecan, Harlem, GA 30814 Worker installing a new compressed air pipe was killed when the pipe exploded and struck his head.*

- *03/03/2012 Tire Centers LLC, Decatur, AL 35601 Worker repairing an off-road tire was killed when the multi-piece rim exploded and struck him.*

- *03/06/2012 Epstein Construction Inc., Chicago, IL 60661 Construction manager driving his truck on worksite suffered an apparent heart aneurism causing him to lose control of vehicle and strike a piece of construction equipment.*

- *03/06/2012 National Steel City LLC, Calvert, AL 36513 Worker installing duct work in building under construction died after falling 60 feet.*

- *03/06/2012 Berlanga General Painting, Eagle Pass, TX 78852 Worker using an aerial lift to paint air ducts died after falling nearly 30 feet from a catwalk.*

- *03/07/2012 Sieveking Inc., Hazelwood, MO 63042 Worker using a portable ladder to hook a hose to a fuel tank truck died after falling 10 feet off the ladder to pavement.*

- *03/08/2012 Nugent's Tree Service Inc., Massapequa, NY 11758 Worker died after falling while trimming trees.* "[36]

As further cited:

"Date of Incident Company and Location Preliminary Description of Incident

- *02/02/2012 Southland Tube Inc., Birmingham, AL 35234 Worker loading steel coils onto an uncoiler died after being found with his head caught between 14,000-pound coils.*

- *02/17/2012 Jackson Pipe & Steel, Leary, TX 75503 Worker operating a jib crane was killed when the steel column supporting the crane fell off its support base causing the column and crane to collapse on him.*

- *02/21/2012 W.A. Felix Builders, Honolulu, HI 96821 Worker died from falling debris while working in a trench.*

- *02/21/2012 Brunner Equipment LLC, Elkin, NC 28621 Worker was killed when a hydraulic lift fell on him.*

- *02/22/2012 AB Construction Inc., Dallas, GA 30157 Worker wearing a horizontal lifeline that was connected to an aircraft hangar under construction was killed when the building collapsed.*

- *02/22/2012 Alabama Forklift & Repair Inc., Clanton, AL 35045 Worker trying to remove the oil filter from underneath a forklift was killed when the jack used to elevate the forklift fell on him.*

- *02/23/2012 Best Foam, Sherman, MS 38869 Worker operating a compactor machine used to pack together cut farm crops died after being caught inside the machine.*

- *02/23/2012 Alltex Steel Inc., Sealy, TX 77474 Worker inside of a scissor lift died when trusses hit the lift, tipping it over.*

- *02/23/2012 Roberson Construction & Land Development, Inc., Gatlinburg, TN 37738 Worker was asphyxiated when an unshored wall collapsed while he was cutting rebar inside of a basin.*

- *02/27/2012 Clanton Masonry, Atlanta, GA 30329 Worker standing on a scaffold platform was killed when a forklift hit the platform, which then hit a building under construction. The worker fell and the building collapsed on him.*

- *02/27/2012 CM Joslin Company Inc., Cleveland, TX 77327 Worker helping to cut down trees was struck and killed by a 55-foot tree being cut by another worker.*

- *02/28/2012 Graftech International, Anmoore, WV 26323 Worker died from abdominal wounds when a part from a metal-cutting machine struck him.*

- *02/28/2012 Jennings Farms, Inc., LaVergne, TN 37086 Worker died after being pinned under the front tire while attempting to stop an unattended moving tractor.*

- *02/29/2012 Flatrolled Steel Inc., Houston, TX 77078 Worker died from injuries when a rail car cover struck his head and crushed his chest.*

- *02/29/2012 Elite Pipeline Services, Odessa, TX 79764 Four workers were hospitalized when a flash fire occurred while they cut bolts off an abandoned pipeline.*

- *02/29/2012 Iron Boss Inc., Houston, TX 77056 Worker putting steel I-beams on blocks was killed when a beam struck his head and chest.*

- *03/01/2012 White Hawk Engineering and Design, Kingfisher, OK 73750 Worker surveying a wheat field was struck and killed by a train as he crossed a railroad track.*

- *03/02/2012 Stein Inc., Ashland, KY 41101 Worker performing machine maintenance was crushed between a conveyor belt and machine frame after an unexpected start-up.*

- *03/02/2012 Ohio American Water, Tiffin, OH 44883 Worker was struck and killed by a vehicle while operating a water valve.*

- *02/29/2012 Elite Pipeline Services, Odessa, TX 79764 Four workers were hospitalized when a flash fire occurred while they cut bolts off an abandoned pipeline.* "[37]

And, as further cited:

"Date of Incident Company and Location Preliminary Description of Incident

- *02/07/2012 Great White Pressure Pumping, Garden City, TX 79739 Worker performing pre-fracking operations was struck and killed when a pipe exploded under pressure.*

- *02/08/2012 Redmond Construction Inc., Bernard, IA 52032 Worker died from head injuries after falling 15 feet while doing construction work.*

- *02/17/2012 US Airways Group Inc., Phoenix, AZ 85034 Worker was crushed between two vertically moving conveyor belts.*

- *02/18/2012 Duphil Construction, Orange, TX 77632 Worker was crushed when a load on a forklift fell.*

- *02/18/2012 Smithfield Packing Company Inc., Clinton, NC 28328 Worker emptying waste water sludge into a tanker truck died from exposure to toxic gas.*

- *02/19/2012 Stevens Pass Mountain Resort, Skyomish, WA 98288 Worker participating in a video shoot at a ski resort was killed during an avalanche.*

- *02/19/2012 Southern Metals Recycling Inc., Savannah, GA 31405 Worker using knife to cut wire cut his finger. He fainted and later died from head injuries after falling to concrete floor.*

- *02/20/2012 CSI Acquistion Co., LLC dba Crane Service Inc., Three Rivers, TX 78022 Worker died when caught between a tractor and a trailer while hooking them together.*

- *02/20/2012 Win-Sons Poleline Construction, Watonga, OK 73040 Worker replacing lightning arresters on electrical lines was electrocuted after touching an energized line.*

- *02/21/2012 Ferman BMW of Palm Harbor, Palm Harbor, FL 34684 Worker died after falling out of a golf cart.*

- *02/22/2012 Renner Construction, Palmetto, GA 30268 Worker performing residential construction died when he fell off the roof, landing on the lower deck.*

- *02/22/2012 Arden and Howe Car Wash Inc., Sacramento, CA 95825 Worker was struck and killed by a vehicle exiting the car wash.*

- *02/23/2012 Neo Corporation, Gatlinburg, TN 37738 Worker was working adjacent to an embankment when it collapsed.*

- *02/23/2012 Walmart, Streetsbooro, OH 44241 Worker unloading a general merchandise truck died from apparent heart attack."*[38]

It's worth citing one more situation [see Appendix 2 cited below]:

"Following a record 53 charges laid against three companies for a 2007 accident that killed two workers at the oilsands work site, the Alberta Federation of Labour blames the provincial government for not being more vigilant to prevent such a tragedy.

Alberta Occupational Health and Safety (OH&S) announced 53 charges yesterday in connection to the April 24, 2007, accident that also injured four other workers, two seriously, at the Canadian Natural Resources Horizon project, about 75 kilometres north of Fort McMurray.

Twenty-nine charges were laid against CNRL, the operator of the Horizon site where the accident occurred. Another 14 charges were laid against contractors SSEC Canada Ltd. and 10 against the Sinopec Shanghai Engineering Company Ltd. The charges included several counts of failing to ensure the health and safety of the workers. Other charges include failing to ensure that a professional engineer prepared and certified drawings and procedures; failing to ensure the roof support structure inside the tank was stable during assembly; failing to ensure that U-bolt type clips used for fastening rope wire were installed properly; and failing to ensure that wire rope being used was safe. The three companies are expected to make their first court appearance June 8 in Fort McMurray."[39]

As further noted:

"*Hong Liang Liu, 33, an electrical engineer, and Genbao Ge, 27, a scaffolder, died after a roof collapsed in a large oil tank where they were working. Both were non-union employees of Sinopec Shanghai Engineering. CNRL had contracted the company to build the tanks in 2006. Liang had been in Canada since September 2006, while Ge arrived in January 2007. Four other Chinese labourers were injured in the collapse. All were temporary labourers.*"[40]

As further cited in the course:

"*Once the accident scene has been roped off, it's important to begin immediately to gather evidence from as many sources as possible during an investigation. One of the biggest challenges you'll face as an investigator is to determine what information is relevant. You want data that will help you determine what happened, how it happened, and why it happened. Identifying items that answer these questions is the purpose of documenting the accident scene.*"[41]

In this regard, as an investigator you should:

"*Make personal observations*

With clipboard in hand, take notes on personal observations. Try to involve all of your senses (sight, hearing, smell, etc.).

What do you see? What equipment, tools, materials, machines, or structures appear to be broken, damaged, struck or otherwise involved in the event? Look for gouges, scratches, dents, smears. If vehicles are involved, check for tracks and skid marks. Look for irregularities on surfaces. Are there any fluid spills, stains, contaminated materials or debris?

What about the environment? Were there any distractions, adverse conditions caused by weather? Record the time of day, location, lighting conditions, etc. Note the terrain (flat, rough, etc.).

What is the activity occurring around the accident scene?

Who is there: Who is not? You'll need this information to take initial statements and interviews.

Measure distances and positions of anything and everything you believe to be of any value to the investigation." [42]

In addition, as cited:

*"**Take photos of the accident scene***

When taking photos, make sure you start with distance shots, and gradually move in closer as you take the photos.

Take video clips of the scene

There is no requirement to take video. However, with the video capability of digital cameras, it's becoming more common to use this method.

Sketch the accident scene

Sketches are very important because they complement the information in photos, and are good at indicating distances between the various elements of the accident. This is important to do because it establishes "position evidence." It is important to be as precise as possible when making sketches." [43]

As further noted:

"Interview records

That's right...you don't just review records, you "interview" them by asking them questions. If you ask...they will answer. Below are some of the records you may want to interview.

- *Maintenance records*
- *Training records*
- *Standard operating procedures*
- *Safety policies, plans, and rules*
- *Work schedules*
- *Personnel records*

- *Disciplinary records*
- *Medical records (if permission granted, or otherwise allowed.)*
- *EMT reports*
- *OSHA 300 Log*
- *OSHA Form 301, Injury and Illness Incident Report*
- *Safety committee minutes*
- *Coroner's report*
- *Police report"* [44]

Footnotes

1 - 3. *Title 29 › Subtitle B › Chapter XVII › Part 1904 › Subpart E › Section 1904.39*
http://www.law.cornell.edu/cfr/text/29/1904.39

4 - 9. *Injury reporting: Tell it to the WCB*
By: Cindy Freiman
2000-10-01
http://www.ohscanada.com/news/injury-reporting-tell-it-to-the-wcb/1000156702/

10 - 13. *WCAT-2009-01297 (Re), 2009 CanLII 36791 (BC WCAT)*
Date: 2009-05-13
Docket: WCAT-2009-01297
http://www.canlii.org/eliisa/highlight.do?text=%22Bill+14%22+prosecutions&language=
en&searchTitle=British+Columbia&path=/en/bc/bcwcat/doc/2009/2009canlii36791/2009
canlii36791.html

14 - 15. *Injury reporting: Tell it to the WCB*
By: Cindy Freiman
2000-10-01
http://www.ohscanada.com/news/injury-reporting-tell-it-to-the-wcb/1000156702/

16 - 21. *R. v. Canadian national railway Co., 2003 CanLII 3056 (MB PC)*
Date: 2003-06-20
Parallel citations: [2004] 1 WWR 357; 175 Man R (2d) 263
http://www.canlii.org/eliisa/highlight.do?text=WCB+fatality+fines&language=en&searc
hTitle=Manitoba&path=/en/mb/mbpc/doc/2003/2003canlii3056/2003canlii3056.html

22. *R. v. Canadian national railway Co., 2003 CanLII 3056 (MB PC)*
Date: 2003-06-20
Parallel citations: [2004] 1 WWR 357; 175 Man R (2d) 263
http://www.canlii.org/eliisa/highlight.do?text=WCB+fatality+fines&language=en&searc
hTitle=Manitoba&path=/en/mb/mbpc/doc/2003/2003canlii3056/2003canlii3056.html

Also see: "*Duties of Employees - Safety and health matters*

126. (1) While at work, every employee shall

(a)   use such safety materials, equipment, devices and clothing as are intended for the employee's protection and furnished to the employee by the employer or as are prescribed;

(b)   follow prescribed procedures with respect to the safety and health of employees;

(c)   take all reasonable and necessary precautions to ensure the safety and health of the employee, the other employees and any person likely to be affected by the employee's acts or omissions;

(d)   comply with all instructions from the employer concerning the safety and health of employees;

(e)   cooperate with any person exercising a duty imposed by this Part or any regulations made thereunder;

(f)   cooperate with the safety and health committee established for the work place where the employee is employed, or if there is no such committee, with the safety and health representative, if any, appointed for that work place;

(g)   report to the employer any thing or circumstances in a work place that is likely to be hazardous to the safety or health of the employee, the other employees or other persons granted access to the work place by the employer;

(h)   report in the manner prescribed every accident or other occurrence arising in the course of or in connection with the employee's work that has caused injury to the employee or to any other person; and

(i)   comply with every oral or written direction of a safety officer concerning the safety and health of employees.

(2) Nothing in subsection (1) relieves an employer from any duty imposed on the employer under this Part."

23 - 24. *R. v. Canadian national railway Co.*, 2003 CanLII 3056 (MB PC)
Date: 2003-06-20
Parallel citations: [2004] 1 WWR 357; 175 Man R (2d) 263
http://www.canlii.org/eliisa/highlight.do?text=WCB+fatality+fines&language=en&searchTitle=Manitoba&path=/en/mb/mbpc/doc/2003/2003canlii3056/2003canlii3056.html

25 - 26. *Title 29 › Subtitle B › Chapter XVII › Part 1904 › Subpart E › Section 1904.39*
http://www.law.cornell.edu/cfr/text/29/1904.39

27 - 34. *R. v. North American Food Produce Byers Ltd., 2006 ONCJ 137 (CanLII)*
Date: 2006-04-13
http://www.canlii.org/eliisa/highlight.do?text=Workplace+Safety+and+Insurance+Act+fa
tality+fines&language=en&searchTitle=Ontario&path=/en/on/oncj/doc/2006/2006oncj13
7/2006oncj137.html

35. *Weekly Reports of Fatalities, Catastrophes, and Other Events*
U.S. Department of Labor, Occupational Safety & Health Administration
http://www.osha.gov/dep/fatcat/dep_fatcat.html

36. *Weekly Summary (Federal and State data tabulated week ending March 10, 2012)*
U.S. Department of Labor, Occupational Safety & Health Administration
http://www.osha.gov/dep/fatcat/fatcat_weekly_rpt_03102012.html

37. *Weekly Summary (Federal and State data tabulated week ending March 3, 2012)*
U.S. Department of Labor, Occupational Safety & Health Administration
http://www.osha.gov/dep/fatcat/fatcat_weekly_rpt_03032012.html

38. *Weekly Summary (Federal and State data tabulated week ending February 25, 2012)*
U.S. Department of Labor, Occupational Safety & Health Administration
http://www.osha.gov/dep/fatcat/fatcat_weekly_rpt_02252012.html

39 - 40. *53 charges for CNRL, Contractors in Deaths of Foreign Workers*
Carol Christian
Today staff
http://oilsandstruth.org/53-charges-cnrl-contractors-deaths-foreign-workers

41 - 44. *702 Accident Investigation*
Steven J. Geigle, MA, CET, CSHM
OSHAcademy Safety and Health Training
www.oshatrain.org

Appendix 2

53 charges for CNRL, Contractors in Deaths of Foreign Workers
Carol Christian
Today staff
http://oilsandstruth.org/53-charges-cnrl-contractors-deaths-foreign-workers

Following a record 53 charges laid against three companies for a 2007 accident that killed two workers at the oilsands work site, the Alberta Federation of Labour blames the provincial government for not being more vigilant to prevent such a tragedy.

Alberta Occupational Health and Safety (OH&S) announced 53 charges yesterday in connection to the April 24, 2007, accident that also injured four other workers, two seriously, at the Canadian Natural Resources Horizon project, about 75 kilometres north of Fort McMurray.

Twenty-nine charges were laid against CNRL, the operator of the Horizon site where the accident occurred. Another 14 charges were laid against contractors SSEC Canada Ltd. and 10 against the Sinopec Shanghai Engineering Company Ltd. The charges included several counts of failing to ensure the health and safety of the workers. Other charges include failing to ensure that a professional engineer prepared and certified drawings and procedures; failing to ensure the roof support structure inside the tank was stable during assembly; failing to ensure that U-bolt type clips used for fastening rope wire were installed properly; and failing to ensure that wire rope being used was safe. The three companies are expected to make their first court appearance June 8 in Fort McMurray.

Hong Liang Liu, 33, an electrical engineer, and Genbao Ge, 27, a scaffolder, died after a roof collapsed in a large oil tank where they were working. Both were non-union employees of Sinopec Shanghai Engineering. CNRL had contracted the company to build the tanks in 2006. Liang had been in Canada since September 2006, while Ge arrived in January 2007. Four other Chinese labourers were injured in the collapse. All were temporary labourers.

No one was injured when a second tank collapsed a few weeks later because the area was still under a stop-work order that covered the three of the 15 tanks from the April 24 accident.

"For the duration of the Horizon project, we maintained a strong safety record on the construction site. We were deeply saddened by the tragic deaths of the two contract workers and the related injuries to the associated contract workers. Our heartfelt sympathies are again extended to their families, friends and co-workers," said CNRL in a statement issued yesterday afternoon.

Through that same statement, the company noted that as the incident is now in "formal legal proceedings," it will issue no further comments until the matter has been resolved.

Meanwhile, the Alberta Federation of Labour says that once it was learned that a company from a Third World country with substandard construction safety history had been contracted to do the work, the government should have immediately stepped in to ensure the safety of the site.

"The government ignored the warning signs," said Gil McGowan, AFL president.

Saying the provincial government dropped the ball, he said when it became public knowledge that CNRL was hiring a Chinese contracting firm to do all the work involved in construction of the tank farm, the provincial government should have stepped in to ensure this company was observing Canadian standards for both worksite safety and construction practices, and not importing substandard Third World practices.

McGowan said it's a company that has had all of its experience in China, which has an abysmal record when it comes to workplace safety especially in the construction industry.

"That fact alone should have been setting off alarm bells for provincial regulators and inspectors. The government should have had its inspectors on that site from Day 1 supervising the project and making sure Canadian practices and rules were being observed," he said. "That didn't happen, and the result was this unprecedented tank collapse, which took the lives of two workers and inured four others." McGowan said this is a tragedy that could have been prevented if the government had seen the red flags and sent inspectors to the site even before ground was broken. Everyone involved in the construction industry knew this was an accident waiting to happen.

"The real tragedy here is that the government ignored the warning signs."

An important lesson from this case, he said, is the government needs to be extra vigilant when it comes to construction companies coming into Canada from abroad that are not familiar with the Canadian construction context and that are not up to speed on Canadian health and safety rules or accepted Canadian construction practices.

"We think that the Chinese contractors' lack of familiarity with Canadian standards and practices is at the root of this tragedy. Frankly, we're concerned that they imported substandard practices along with their management team."

Though he's pleased the government is proceeding with charges against the companies involved, McGowan said he's "troubled" over the time it took and is concerned Crown prosecutors "dragged their heels."

"We think what happened on the CNRL site was one of the most serious violations of occupational health and safety rules and standards that we've seen in this province in a

long time, and this is clearly a case where the companies involved have to be held to account," said McGowan, acknowledging it was satisfying to see the charges hadn't forgotten the injured workers. Some of the charges, all laid under the Occupational Health and Safety Act, also take into account the injured workers and the severity of their injuries as well as workers present when the accident occurred.

But the bigger concern for the AFL is that it's not convinced the charges are enough to prevent a another incident. The only way to avoid such a repeat is if the provincial government becomes more serious about enforcing its own health and safety rules, especially on construction worksites before accidents happen instead of waiting until after someone has died.

"Despite the number of charges being laid, it will be the courts that will determine the facts of the case, and determine the appropriate penalties, if any," said Barrie Harrison, OH&S spokesman, yesterday. The OH&S Act allows for up to a maximum $500,000 fine for each charge.

It's expected the Crown will only move ahead on those charges that carry a reasonable likelihood of conviction, Harrison said.

"Whether it's 53 charges or one, Occupational Health and Safety takes workplace health and safety extremely seriously and whether it's an injury on site or a death, or in this case a double fatality, all are taken seriously. I think our record over the last number of years when it comes to the number of charges and prosecutions have proven that."

When a workplace accident — fatal or not — occurs, OH&S has two years to lay charges. In this case, charges came three days shy of the deadline.

The investigation takes a number of months and is followed by a review of the file and work with Crown prosecutors to determine what charges, if any, are warranted.

"It's that process that takes a fair bit of time," said Harrison. More important, he added, OH&S had to ensure this investigation was proper and thorough because it was focusing on the loss of two lives.

"At the end of the day, that's probably the most important thing. To us, of course, regardless of where these workers are from, their place of origin, or country of birth, has no bearing, because every worker in Alberta has to be treated the same, and these are people who have friends and families and co-workers like the rest of us, and they deserve nothing less."

During the OH&S investigation, Alberta Employment and Immigration determined that 132 Chinese temporary foreign workers were not paid from April to July 2007. Their employer was SSEC Canada, and it is yet not clear why they weren't paid.

As a result, CNRL transferred $3.17 million to the province within the past couple of months for distribution to these workers.

"These funds are now held in a government trust account and we've begun the process of verifying individuals' identity and establishing a process for the distribution of these unpaid earnings," said Harrison. "We want to make sure that we do exercise all due diligence to ensure that these are getting directly in the hands of those who deserve it."

Meanwhile, he said the province will make "every reasonable effort" to collect the money from SSEC. If successful, CNRL will be reimbursed accordingly, he added.

Chapter 8 – "The harmful transfer of energy is the direct cause of injury"

As cited in our OH&S course, "the harmful transfer of energy is the direct cause of injury"[1], which can be analyzed by looking at:

- *Direct cause of injury*
- *Surface cause of the accident*
- *Root cause of the accident*
- *Injury analysis*
- *Surface cause analysis*
- Root cause analysis[2]

As further cited:

"It's important to understand that all injuries to workers are caused by one thing: the harmful transfer of energy. Let's take a look at some examples that illustrate this important principle.

If a harsh acid splashes on your face, you may suffer a chemical burn because your skin has been exposed to a chemical form of energy that destroys tissue. In this instance, the direct cause of the injury is a harmful chemical reaction. The related surface causes might be the acidic nature of the chemical (condition) and working without proper face protection (unsafe behavior).

If your workload is to too strenuous, force requirements on your body may cause a muscle strain. Here, the direct cause of injury is a harmful level of kinetic energy (energy resulting from motion), causing injury to muscle tissue. A related surface cause of the accident might be fatigue (hazardous condition) or improper lifting techniques (unsafe behavior).

The important point to remember here is that the "direct cause" of the injury is not the same as the "surface cause" of the accident event.

The direct cause of injury is the harmful transfer of energy as a consequence of your exposure to that energy. The direct result of this harmful energy transfer is injury.

The surface cause of the accident is the condition or behavior that interact in a way that results in the harmful transfer of energy." [3]

Let's look at some of these factors.

In terms of a harmful transfer of energy, as referenced in Rockett (1998), it was mentioned:

"In the 1960s, psychologist James Gibson specified that physical energy was the agent in the epidemiologic triad of injuries - enabling a great 'etiologic leap' in injury research."[4]

"Injury can occur when our capacity to control energy is compromised, such as when a person falls asleep while driving, or when task demands exceed our capacity to control energy, such as when someone swims into a riptide or drives onto an ice patch."[5]

"Too much or too little energy can harm the body. Injury occurs when the release and transfer of energy exceeds the injury threshold. The injury threshold is the point at which the body cannot tolerate the transfer without damage or when energy flows are suppressed below levels necessary for normal functioning."[6]

"All five forms of physical energy - electricity, kinetic energy, chemical energy, thermal energy, and radiation - are injury agents."[7]

With respect to radiation injury, it is noted "radiation injuries are caused by ionizing radiation emitted by sources such as the sun, x-ray and other diagnostic machines, tanning beds, and radioactive elements released in nuclear power plant accidents and detonation of nuclear weapons during war and as terrorist acts."[8]

A brief description, "ionizing radiation is made up of unstable atoms that contain an excess amount of energy. In an attempt to stabilize, the atoms emit the excess energy into the atmosphere, creating radiation. Radiation can either be electromagnetic or particulate."[9]

With:

"Any amount of ionizing radiation will produce some damage … Radiation can damage every tissue in the body. The particular manifestation will depend upon the amount of radiation, the time over which it is absorbed, and the susceptibility of the tissue. The fastest growing tissues are the most vulnerable, because radiation as much as triples its effects during the growth phase. Bone marrow cells that make blood are the fastest growing cells in the body. A fetus in the womb is equally sensitive. The germinal cells in the testes and ovaries are only slightly less sensitive. Both can be rendered useless with very small doses of radiation. More resistant are the lining cells of the body—skin and intestines. Most resistant are the brain cells, because they grow the slowest." [10]

Direct cause of injury

In terms of a direct cause of injury, one has to establish this to be fact. In this case[11], the appeal involved:

"[1]   This is an appeal of a decision from the Dispute Resolution and Decision Review Body (DRDRB) which determined that the worker did not have an acceptable claim for coverage from the Workers' Compensation Board (WCB).

[2]   The worker filed a claim with the WCB indicating that the performance of his regular work duties caused him to suffer a personal injury to his knees. The WCB ultimately decided that the worker did not have an acceptable claim and the worker asked the DRDRB to review this decision.

[3]   The DRDRB reviewed the worker's claim and in a decision dated November 24, 2010 upheld the findings of the WCB and determined that the worker did not have an acceptable claim for coverage from the WCB. The worker appealed and notice of his appeal was received by the Appeals Commission on December 3, 2010."[12]

The worker had filed a claim that:

"[4]   The worker filed a Worker's Report of Injury on March 2, 2010 claiming that his work duties caused extreme strain on his knees which in turn caused him to suffer a bilateral injury to his knees."[13]

And, the worker appealed this decision:

"[6]   At the worker's request the DRDRB reviewed his file. The DRDRB found that the worker's knee injury was neither directly caused by his work duties nor did he suffer an "aggravation" in accordance with WCB Policy 03-02 Part II. The DRDRB upheld the WCB's decision and concluded that the worker did not have an acceptable claim for WCB coverage."[14]

The issue for this court was:

"[8]   Does the worker have an acceptable Workers' Compensation Board claim for a bilateral injury to his knees?"[15]

The pertinent worker submissions included:

"[20]   The worker's representative (representative) and the worker provided submissions which we have summarized as follows:

[20.1]   The worker commenced working for the employer in September, 2007. In June, 2009 he started to notice pain in his knees and attended upon a general physician to seek treatment.

[20.2]   The worker continued to work for the employer and his duties did not change. The worker's knees continued to worsen until he was no long able to perform his regular job duties.

[20.3]   The worker believes that the physically demanding nature of job duties caused the injury to his knees. This belief is supported by the weight of medical evidence.

[20.4]   The worker has concerns regarding the assessment of his critical job demands. He does not feel that the WCB case manager or the person conducting the assessment truly appreciated the physical nature of his job. Further that in conducting the assessment the WCB relied too heavily on the employer's suggestion that the worker's duties were significantly less demanding than stated by the worker.

[20.5]   In any event, the critical job demands summary still found that the worker was required to use a manual pallet jack on a regular basis. This work caused the worker to perform at least occasional dynamic pushing and pulling of pallets weighing up to 3400 pounds."[16]

With the court mentioning "in order for the worker's claim to be accepted, all that needs to be found is that there was a causal relationship between his work duties and the injuries to his knees. The weight of evidence supports that either the worker's job duties directly caused him to suffer injuries to his knees or that he suffered an aggravation to a pre-existing condition and consequently the worker should be entitled to WCB coverage."[17]

With this court highlighting previous findings:

"[25]   We find that the weight of evidence does not support that there is a direct causal relationship between the worker's knee symptoms and his work duties. We make this finding based on the following evidence and for the following reasons:

[25.1]   The WCB arranged for the worker to take part in a Return to Work Services assessment which included a medical status examination (MSE). The worker was examined by a WCB physician (MSE physician) on May 3, 2010 who provided a diagnosis of "possible bilateral degenerative medial meniscal tears" and recommended that an expedited magnetic resonance imaging (MRI) scan of the worker's knees take place.

[25.2]   A MRI scan of the worker's knees was performed on May 3, 2010. The corresponding report contained the following findings:

"LEFT KNEE Impression:

Horizontal cleavage tear with the posterior horn and body of the medial meniscus as described above.

RIGHT KNEE Impression:

1.   Comminuted full thickness tear of the posterior horn of the medial meniscus of the right knee as described above. ...

2.   Mild chondromalacia patellae."[18]

Continuing with:

"[25.3]   The WCB arranged to have the worker's file reviewed by a WCB medical consultant (medical consultant). In a report dated August 24, 2010 the medical consultant made the following comments and provided the following opinion:

On April 21, 2010, a Critical Job Demand Summary was completed. It indicated that the worker believed that his heavy lifting and pushing and pulling of the pallet jack was responsible for the strain on his knees bilaterally. ... The worker claimed that on occasion he had to pull the pallet jack into the warehouse. Reportedly many of the products weighed up to 2000 pounds on the pallet. ...

1.   Please confirm the diagnosis affecting the left and right knee.

This writer is of the opinion that [the MSE physician's diagnosis on May 3, 2010 of bilateral degenerative medial meniscal tears is correct. This was supported by the MRI scan of both knees which revealed degenerative tears of both medial menisci. ... Both knees had joint effusions compatible with degeneration.

2.   Did the established work activity or exposure contribute to, cause or have significant effect on the condition?

No.

As previously pointed out the worker's knee pain is activity related and that the worker would experience pain in the knees with any activity whether occupational or non-occupational. The worker had been performing his current job duties for 2.5 years and it is not reasonable to attribute the findings on the MRI scan to the worker's job activities as explained by the worksite visit as well as Physical Demands Analysis, Worker's Progressive Injury Questionnaire, and Employer's Progressive Injury Questionnaire.

Judging by the clinical presentation on the MRI scan, this writer is of the opinion that this is further evidence of degenerative tears rather than work-related injuries."[19]

However, the current court in reviewing this material came to a different conclusion, with their decision simply allowing the worker's appeal of this earlier ruling:

"[35]   The worker has an acceptable Workers' Compensation Board claim for a bilateral injury to his knees on the basis of an aggravation factor.

[36]   *The appeal is allowed.*"[20]

Surface cause of the accident

The hazardous conditions and unsafe behaviors we identify as contributing to the accident are called the surface causes of the accident.[21]

As reported, "the surface cause of accidents includes those hazardous conditions and individual unsafe behaviors that directly caused or contributed in some way to the accident."[22]

As further noted, hazardous conditions may exist in any of the following:

- *Materials*
- *Machinery*
- *Equipment*
- *Tools*
- *Chemicals*
- *Environment*
- *Workstations*
- *Facilities*

- *People*
- *Workload*[23]

And, examples of unsafe behaviors may include:

- *Failing to comply with rules*
- *Using unsafe methods*
- *Taking shortcuts*
- *Horseplay*
- *Failing to report injuries*
- *Failing to report hazards*
- *Allowing unsafe behaviors*
- *Failing to train*
- *Failing to supervise*
- *Failing to correct*
- *Scheduling too much work*
- *Ignoring worker stress*[24]

In this court case[25], horseplay was examined as the cause of injury and the consequences thereof.

As cited:

"[1]   On April 21, 2008, the worker submitted a Worker's Report of Injury to the Workers' Compensation Board (WCB) for a left knee injury that occurred at work on April 18, 2008.

[2]   After a period of investigation, the WCB denied the worker's claim for compensation on the basis that his left knee injury did not arise out of his employment. Rather, the WCB decided that the worker's left knee injury occurred as a result of horseplay for which the worker was the instigator. Therefore, he had removed himself from the course of his employment. This decision was communicated to the worker in a letter dated May 6, 2008.

[3]   The worker disagreed with the WCB decision to deny his claim and the matter was then referred to the Dispute Resolution and Decision Review Body (DRDRB) for review."[26]

In the lower decision, the worker's horseplay removed him from employee status as cited:

"[4]   The DRDRB decision of May 29, 2009 stated, in part:

"By Policy 02-01 Part ll, compensation is not payable if the worker's actions at the time of accident have, in the WCB's opinion, removed the worker from the course of employment. The Policy sets out that horseplay, if the worker is the instigator and it is an abandonment of employment duties, is considered to have removed the worker from the course of employment.

I accept that the incident occurred on employer premises during work hours. But, I do not find the conduct of [the worker] was related to employment responsibilities with [the employer], or that the injury occurred from an employment hazard. I find the conduct was horseplay, with [the worker] as the instigator, with no intervening circumstance in the events of the horseplay. I believe [the worker's] conduct was with a wanton and reckless disregard of probable consequences and his conduct removed from [sic] himself [from] the course of employment."[27]

The issue for the appeal court was, "what is considered a deviation which removes a worker from the course of employment?"[28]

As further cited:

"When a worker voluntarily engages in an act which is not reasonably expected in the course of employment and which results in abandonment of employment duties, it may be considered a serious deviation. Each case has to be judged on its own merits."[29]

"For example, if a worker walks over to chat with a co-worker and accompanies this with a flicking of elastic bands, it is a trivial incident and would probably be an insubstantial deviation. Similarly, attending to activities of personal comfort that are essential to human needs may be considered incidental to the employment and likely not a deviation."[30]

"However, if a worker plays a joke which requires a significant part of the working time and concentration of energies to the extent that the employment duties are neglected, it may be considered a substantial deviation. Activities such as transacting personal business or going to places that have nothing to do with employment may remove the worker from the course of employment."[31]

The appeal court also had to consider, "is it compensable when horseplay (rough play) resulted in an injury?"[32]

With, "a worker who is injured through instigating or participating in horseplay is not necessarily barred from compensation. The circumstances surrounding the horseplay must be thoroughly reviewed to determine if there is a significant deviation from the course of employment."[33]

Also:

"An injury may still be considered to have arisen out of and in the course of employment if:

- *the interruption of productive activity is too brief to be considered a substantial deviation from the course of employment*

- *the horseplay is a common occurrence at work and is condoned by the employer*

- *the horseplay is initially harmless then escalates into a dangerous activity, and the worker is not a willing participant in the escalation*

- *the worker is still participating in productive activity, or some other activity of the employment even though the task was performed in an un-business-like manner."[34]*

The key submissions by the worker included:

"[18]   The worker and his representative provided submissions which are summarized as follows:

[18.1]   There was no interruption in the productivity at the workplace as the whole incident only took about two minutes at best. It was explained that the incident occurred

after a long coffee break and the workers were on their way back to the work bays to resume repair work on a truck.

[18.2]   Horseplay was a common occurrence at this work site and while there is no specific evidence that the employer condoned horseplay, it is argued that this can be assumed because there was no disciplinary action taken and horseplay often involved participation by the supervisors.

[18.3]   This was initially an innocent prank that was not intended to harm anyone. The worker simply kneeled down behind a co-worker, knowing that a third co-worker would likely tip/push the other co-worker over top of him. The incident escalated when the other two co-workers began to shove and push each other, at which time the worker turned and walked away. This is evidence that it was not the worker who escalated the incident.

[18.4]   The worker's representative stated that when the worker turned his back and walked away, one of his co-workers grabbed him by the shoulder and kneed him in back of his left knee. Therefore, it is argued that it was this co-worker who escalated the situation, and by doing so, caused serious injury to the worker's left knee.

[18.5]   The remedy sought is for this left knee injury to be considered compensable on the basis that although it was caused by horseplay initiated by the worker, he was not a willing participant in the escalation of the situation.[35]

The appeal court ruled:

"[30]   Based on the findings and evidence referenced above, we conclude that the circumstances surrounding the horseplay do not amount to a significant deviation from the expectations and conditions of the worker's employment so as to remove him from the course of his employment. The criteria under Application 5 of Policy 02-01 have been met. Therefore, the worker's left knee injury is considered to have arisen out of and in the course of his employment."[36]

Again with their decision simply allowing the worker's appeal of this earlier ruling:

"[31]   We have decided that the worker's left knee injury did arise out of and occur during the course of his employment. Therefore, the worker has an acceptable claim for compensation.

[32]   The May 29, 2009 Dispute Resolution and Decision Review Body decision is reversed and the worker's appeal is granted."[37]

Root cause of the accident

As further reported, "after we identify surface causes, we'll need to determine if inadequate safety system components contributed to the accident by allowing the hazardous conditions and unsafe behaviors to develop or occur. These system inadequacies are called the root causes of accidents."[38]

And:

"The root causes for accidents are the underlying safety system weaknesses that have somehow contributed to the existence of hazardous conditions and unsafe behaviors that represent surfaces causes of accidents."[39]

With:

"It's important to understand that root causes always pre-exist surface causes. Indeed, inadequately designed system components have the potential to feed and nurture hazardous conditions and unsafe behaviors. If root causes are left unchecked, surface causes will flourish!"[40]

As further reported:

"One of the most important aspects of accident investigation is determining the underlying causes of the accident. Often, people stop the investigation too early, forgetting that each main cause may have several underlying causes. For example, if a person slips on a wet floor and injures themselves, some people would say the 'cause' of the accident was the wet floor. This is correct, but we say this is the IMMEDIATE CAUSE."[41]

"What is more important are the underlying causes, or ROOT CAUSES. For example, what caused the water to be left lying on the floor, did the water come from a leak, had the water been lying on the floor for several minutes or several hours – or even days – before the accident?"[42]

"These questions, and of course their answers, are more beneficial than the actual immediate cause itself. We can learn more about the safety culture of an organisation by investigating root causes, than we can by any other means. Therefore, carrying out an in-depth investigation, which goes beyond the immediate cause, is not only essential; it is very beneficial in the long-term."[43]

Here's another court case[44] that highlights the need for a direct causal link to the injury.

As cited, the case involved:

"[1]   The issue is whether the worker has initial entitlement for her bilateral shoulders.

[2]   The worker, who was born on July 4, 1973, began working as an assembler for the employer a manufacturer of electrical parts on September 18, 1998. She laid off work as a result of a miscarriage in November 1999 and was rehired on December 14, 1999.

[3]   She did not work before immigrating to Canada from India in 1995. After taking English language classes, she began her first job, placing labels on products on a part time basis.

[4]   The worker testified that prior to joining the employer she had experienced no injuries and had no physical problems. In particular she had no shoulder problems. She was 4 feet six inches tall and weighed 85 pounds.

[5]   The worker's first job with the employer was described as "assembly" which required her to reach forward and retrieve plastic housings and wires from bins on her work station. She would insert four wires into receptacles in one side of the housing and then insert four wires on the other side of the housing in the same manner. She would then pull on each wire, with one hand on the housing and the other hand on the wire end in turn, to ensure that the connections were secure.

[6]   The worker testified that initially two people worked on the assembly job and produced 1200 pieces or production harnesses a day and when she started doing it alone she had a target of 800 pieces a day. To produce 800 pieces she had to push to insert a wire and pull to ensure it was properly fastened, 5,120 times a day, as 8 pushes times 8 pulls times 800 pieces equals 5,120. The worker testified that she had to push hard on the wires to insert them and pull hard on them to be certain that they were properly connected with the housing. Because she was diminutive, she had to hold the wire and the housing at the level of her upper chest to apply enough force to properly insert the wire and to test the connection."[45]

The worker attributed her shoulder problems to her job:

"[7]   She originally felt pain in her right shoulder in September 1999 and reported it to her family doctor, Dr. K. Thakkar. Dr. Thakkar ordered an x-ray of both of her shoulders and an x-ray report dated July 27, 2000, revealed no abnormalities in either shoulder.

[8]   In a report dated August 13, 2001, Dr. Thakkar noted that he first saw the worker for right shoulder tendonitis on September 9, 1999 and at the time the worker advised that her job was "pulling wire." He prescribed painkillers. Dr. Thakkar further noted that he subsequently saw the worker for right shoulder problems

on June 25, 2000, July 27, 2000, September 16, 2000 and October 12, 2000. He added that worker had no previous history of shoulder pain that he was aware of."[46]

With the lower decision including this logic:

"The task of pulling on the wires when performing initial assembly and rework is a bilateral task. As the right shoulder is externally rotated to generate tension, the left shoulder must also externally rotate to apply an equal but opposite resistance. If this activity were the root cause of the injury, one would also expect to see similar changes in the non-dominant left shoulder. To my knowledge, there were no reports of a left shoulder injury at the time of my involvement in [the worker's] claim."[47]

In this case, the review panel found:

"[35]   The Panel finds that the worker has initial entitlement for both of her shoulders as a result of her work duties with the accident employer.

[36]   There is no evidence that the worker had experienced any injuries or physical problems before joining the accident employer.

[37]   In the opinion of the Panel, the ergonomist and the ARO misunderstood the mechanics of the way the worker was forced to perform her duties and the impact it had on her shoulders.

[38]   The worker asserted that to ensure that the wires were securely attached to the plastic housings she had to push hard to insert them into the receptacles on the housing and pull hard on the wires to test that that attachment was secure. Otherwise they might come off. The worker was clear in her statements that it was for that reason the job was physically demanding. To use enough force to do the testing she had to hold the housing and the wire at the level of her upper chest and pull very hard.

[39]   The ergonomist did not indicate whether he actually inserted wires into the receptacles on the housings but he did test the wires by pulling them. As he did not appear to know that you had to pull hard on them to ensure they were properly attached, he would have thought he was properly testing by, as he said, asserting minimum force.

[40]   He also would not have understood, (as was pointed out by the worker's representative in his July 4, 2003 submission) that a woman of diminutive stature (4' 6" tall, weighing 85 pounds) would have had to use an exaggerated posture and a hard pull to do her job.

[41] *For this reason, the Panel finds that in doing the assembly job and then briefly the rework job, the worker would have asserted enough force in postures at the level of her upper chest to have, over time, injured both of her shoulders.*

[42] *In the opinion of the Panel, the Board also underestimated the number of repetitive motions the worker would perform in the assembly job. The ergonomist calculated that, using the employer's estimate of the worker completing 600 harnesses a shift, the worker would complete a harness every 78 seconds. Based on a 1994 study indicating that a worker would have to perform 2.5 shoulder movements or contractions a minute to be at risk for shoulder injury, the ergonomist concluded the worker's job was not sufficiently repetitive to put the worker's shoulders at risk.*

[43] *In the Panel's opinion, the worker performed a shoulder movement or contraction each time she pushed or pulled on a wire. As every completed harness required 8 pushes and 8 pulls in the slightly over a minute it took to produce a harness, the worker would perform well in excess of 2.5 shoulder movements or contractions a minute and therefore be at risk over time for shoulder injuries.*

[44] *One of the reasons given by the ergonomist for excluding the worker's job duties as a cause of her shoulders problems was that "if this activity were the root cause of the injury one would also expect to see similar changes in the non-dominant left shoulder." According to the ergonomist "there were no reports of a left shoulder injury at the time of my involvement in [the worker's] claim." There is, in fact, ample evidence of a contemporaneous left shoulder problem."*[48]

With a final disposition of:

"[52] *The appeal is allowed.*

[53] *The worker has initial entitlement for her bilateral shoulders.*

[54] *The Board shall determine the nature and extent of the benefits that flow from this decision."*[49]

Footnotes

1 – 3. *702 Accident Investigation*
Steven J. Geigle, MA, CET, CSHM
OSHAcademy Safety and Health Training
www.oshatrain.org

4 - 7. Ian R.H. Rockett. "Injury and Violence: A Public Health Perspective", *Population Bulletin*, 53(4), December, 1998
https://docs.google.com/viewer?a=v&q=cache:PwN2-32IIOcJ:www.prb.org/source/53.4injuryviolence.pdf+harmful+transfer+of+energy+is+th

e+direct+cause+of+injury&hl=en&gl=ca&pid=bl&srcid=ADGEESiK7KAXmBtSoBvp8
bxd0p0FQMu3kNMNhCtWmsTfzsKXqe1hE4unBqgJYhoxuNhetKY7iXL5TJapwjY_sF
ciCgoNT4XU0CLkgPAOJgkJpXSxXE4x7g0WgAgbC6Fsw71RixnV-
0Yn&sig=AHIEtbQ1eNCaLFOO6vx8OwLKChpI0aTNcg

8 – 10. *Radiation Injuries*
http://medical-dictionary.thefreedictionary.com/Radiation+Injuries

11 - 20. *Decision No: 2011-909, 2011 CanLII 62782 (AB WCAC)*
Date: 2011-10-07
Docket: 2011-909; 43415
http://www.canlii.org/eliisa/highlight.do?text=Direct+cause+of+injury+to+workers&lang
uage=en&searchTitle=Search+all+CanLII+Databases&path=/en/ab/abwcac/doc/2011/20
11canlii62782/2011canlii62782.html

21. *Fixing the System with Root Cause Analysis*, Oregon Occupational Safety and Health
Division (Oregon OSHA), Salem, Oregon, USA.
https://docs.google.com/viewer?a=v&q=cache:Su7ajLYNBvsJ:apps.ocfl.net/dept/county
_admin/public_safety/risk/modrootcause.pdf+%22Surface+cause%22+of+workers+accid
ent&hl=en&gl=uk&pid=bl&srcid=ADGEESgSzJ-
4JUj8Qnq8HuW6n_VkOVYtU63_xfJSYVvU6H3K72wHFYPFx5lTsxRbAT6b4-
3TRuZ8Dof_U_WE1Ws3RzM2JmITnoZT16HwkCAlHNrD-
Rc7YJ8arNcFZk_Cmbn6YZz6xgUB&sig=AHIEtbTWj7oCsLv8a9lZkrf31S3lqeR_Nw

22 - 24. *ILLINOIS INSTITUTE OF TECHNOLOGY SAFETY COMMITTEE: INCIDENT
INVESTIGATION POLICY AND INVESTIGATION FORM*
Approved: June 19, 2006
https://docs.google.com/viewer?a=v&q=cache:_PDpBC6zJeYJ:www.iit.edu/general_cou
nsel/pdfs/incident_invest_policy.pdf+Surface+cause+of+worker's+accident&hl=en&gl=c
a&pid=bl&srcid=ADGEESgDEG0bMsm1Rslm8gs51ubMFkZZGtSYZ71hlghU9aKUsX
SmwbEMClmdJcKoxCYW2bZjNRQ60Onb_hS-
U899AyU9WOdZTRQRy3Gh97SFvWkletwpidlLddya48YI10-
sAw2xAejS&sig=AHIEtbQh64COflfplDZWAzSnTU7VIDlQ1w

25 - 37. *Decision No.: 2009-1013, 2009 CanLII 63797 (AB WCAC)*
Date: 2009-11-06
Docket: 39499; 2009-1013
http://www.canlii.org/eliisa/highlight.do?text=Horseplay+cause+of+injury+to+workers&
language=en&searchTitle=Search+all+CanLII+Databases&path=/en/ab/abwcac/doc/200
9/2009canlii63797/2009canlii63797.html

38 - 40. *Fixing the System with Root Cause Analysis*, Oregon Occupational Safety and
Health Division (Oregon OSHA), Salem, Oregon, USA.
https://docs.google.com/viewer?a=v&q=cache:Su7ajLYNBvsJ:apps.ocfl.net/dept/county
_admin/public_safety/risk/modrootcause.pdf+%22Surface+cause%22+of+workers+accid

ent&hl=en&gl=uk&pid=bl&srcid=ADGEESgSzJ-
4JUj8Qnq8HuW6n_VkOVYtU63_xfJSYVvU6H3K72wHFYPFx5lTsxRbAT6b4-
3TRuZ8Dof_U_WE1Ws3RzM2JmITnoZT16HwkCAlHNrD-
Rc7YJ8arNcFZk_Cmbn6YZz6xgUB&sig=AHIEtbTWj7oCsLv8a9lZkrf31S3lqeR_Nw

41 - 43. *How to Investigate an Accident at Work*
Author: Norman Thomson - Updated: 3 October 2010
Workplace Safety Advice
http://www.workplacesafetyadvice.co.uk/investigate-accident-work.html

44 - 49. *Decision No. 684/09, 2009 ONWSIAT 1125 (CanLII)*
Date: 2009-05-06
Docket: 684/09
http://www.canlii.org/eliisa/highlight.do?text=Root+cause+of+injury+to+workers&langu
age=en&searchTitle=Search+all+CanLII+Databases&path=/en/on/onwsiat/doc/2009/200
9onwsiat1125/2009onwsiat1125.html

Chapter 9 – "What is a good recommendation?"

As cited in our OH&S course:

An accident investigation is generally thought to be a "reactive" safety process because it is initiated only after an accident has occurred. However, if we propose recommendations that include effective immediate corrective actions and system improvements, we may transform the investigation into a valuable "proactive" process that helps to prevent future injuries.[1]

In a report to the Ministry of Labour in Ontario, Canada[2] it was cited:

"If this report is fully implemented, every Ontario worker and supervisor will receive mandatory information about workplace rights and responsibilities before they start their job; every construction worker will receive entry-level training on construction site safety; there will be rigorous training standards for workers who work at heights and on other high risk activities there will be tougher penalties for those who place workers at risk of death or serious injury; employers will receive better support in understanding and meeting health and safety standards and greater recognition where these are exceeded; the needs and realities of operating small businesses will be accommodated in labour policies; there will be a renewed prevention organization with focused leadership heading a more integrated, efficient and accountable system; and there will be more information and better protection available for vulnerable workers."[3]

With "more open and transparent consultation with the workplace parties coupled with these and other recommendations in this report will assist you in promoting safer and healthier workplaces"[4] [see Appendix 3 cited below].

In terms of union and employer co-operation when it comes to safety, the following was cited in this case:

a)   *The Employer and the Union agree that they mutually desire to maintain standards of safety and health in the Hospital in order to prevent accidents, injury and illness.*

b)   *Recognizing its responsibilities under the applicable legislation, the Hospital agrees to accept as a member of its Occupational Health & Safety Committee at least one (1) representative selected or appointed by the Union from amongst bargaining unit employees.*

c)   *Such Committee shall identify potential dangers and hazards, institute means of improving health and safety programs and recommend actions to be taken to improve conditions related to safety and health.*

d)   The Hospital agrees to co-operate reasonably in providing necessary information to enable the Committee to fulfill its functions.

e)   Meetings shall be held every second month or more frequently at the call of the chair if required. The Committee shall maintain minutes of all meetings and make the same available for review.

f)   Any representative appointed or selected in accordance with 20.02 hereof shall serve for a term of one (1) calendar year from the date of appointment which may be renewed for further periods of one (1) year. Time off for such representative(s) to attend meetings of the Occupational Health & Safety Committee in accordance with the foregoing shall be granted and any representative(s) attending such meetings during their regularly scheduled hours of work shall not lose regular earnings as a result of such attendance.

g)   The Union agrees to endeavour to obtain the full cooperation of its membership in the observation of all safety rules and practices.[5]

Occupational Health & Safety even continues after accident or injury.

As cited in this case[6]:

"Under the Act, the Commission may pursue rehabilitation under the provisions of section 43. That section reads:

43   To aid in getting injured workers back to work and to assist in lessening or removing any handicap resulting from their injuries, the Commission may take such measures and make such expenditures as it may deem necessary or expedient, and the expense thereof shall be borne and may be collected in the same manner as compensation or expenses of administration."[7]

With an extension to include:

"The extent of section 43 was recently interpreted in the case of Fundy Linen Services Inc. v. Workplace Health, Safety and Compensation Commission, 2009 NBCA 13 (CanLII), 2009 NBCA 13 (CanLII). The Court in that case stated at paragraph 47 of its decision:

...Section s. 43 of the Act vests the Commission with a discretionary power to make expenditures the Commission deems advisable. While it is under no legal obligation to provide injured workers with housing alternatives, as a matter of discretion and policy it has decided to do so. However, entitlement is subject to the Commission's Policy Directive. In turn, that directive sets down a number of matters that must be examined before a decision respecting financial assistance is made...."[8]

However, psychological care must be tied to physical / vocational rehabilitation:

"Ms. [the appellant] was transferred to this writer for ongoing psychological services focused on dealing with anxiety, depression, chronic pain and workplace harassment. She notes some progress from her counseling services thus far, however admits that at the beginning she primarily needed to debrief regarding the workplace incident. She continues to ruminate excessively regarding this incident and is quite determined to continue to pursue this matter. We have mostly focused during our 4 therapy sessions on establishing therapeutic rapport and understanding her current situation ...

the Appeals Tribunal accepts the appellant's appeal as it relates to the provision of psychological care and, to this extent, the appeal is accepted. However, the Appeals Tribunal does not accept that the appellant is unable to participate in her vocational rehabilitation program which the Commission has proposed. Her benefits were by reason of her lack of participation properly suspended and will remain suspended pending her return to the rehabilitation program."[9]

An important factor to workplace health and safety, as cited, includes: "several studies show that workplaces with better trained committee members tend to have good health and safety records."[10]

In fact:

"Experience with joint committees appears to have convinced many employers that these committees can play a useful role in reducing accidents and improving safety - and that management does not lose control of the workplace."[11]

"The Ontario survey, for example, noted that 66.9 percent of managers and 60.3percent of workers generally agreed that their committee had achieved the stated goal of "equal" influence by both parties."[12]

"Nevertheless, it also concluded that managers tended to have more influence on committees than workers."[13]

"Management ultimately retained the power to implement JHSC recommendations."[14]

"While management was required to discuss decisions with the joint committees, it also had wide discretion over what decisions it felt were appropriate for committee discussion."[15]

"The study also noted that management representatives on joint committees had closer links to ministry inspectors and the enforcement agencies."[16]

"Finally, it was noted that management representatives were, for the most part, better trained and more knowledgeable on health and safety issues and legislation than most worker representatives (Ontario Advisory Council 1986, 69-81)."[17]

However, employee participation is important in such committees:

"Joint OH&S Committees are one way that workers exercise their right to participate."[18]

"Workers are knowledgeable about the OH&S concerns in their workplaces and how to fix them."[19]

"It's through Joint OH&S Committees that workers have input into solutions that make their workplaces safer and healthier."[20]

Unfortunately, young workers seem to be left out:

"We recently surveyed a group of young workers regarding on-the-job occupational health and safety training. By 'training,' we mean formal training sessions on safety risks, risk management and supervision within the workplace."[21]

"More specifically, our goal was to ascertain from the respondents if their employer or supervisor provided OHS training before they took up their jobs or during their first week of work. Only 40% of the youth said their employer took the initiative to provide training."[22]

"In other words, three out of five of the young workers received no OHS training when they started their jobs."[23]

Also reported in this study:

"How do young people react when their safety at work is at risk? The study revealed that some young workers would react to an unsafe situation before a potential accident, some wouldn't react, and others would react after running the risk."[24]

"Thirty-nine percent would continue working as though nothing was wrong but would later talk about it with friends or colleagues, while 11% would continue working but would later call a government official to complain. These young workers run the risk and subsequently seek intervention."[25]

This case[26] exemplifies this unfortunate aspect with young workers.

At paragraphs 8 and 11, it is cited:

[8]   In mitigation of its culpability I acknowledge that the defendant had a safety program in place. It did conduct an orientation and brief training of the young worker which I found to be cursory in its nature. [27]

[11]   The aggravating factors, as will be clear from my judgment in this matter, arise from the failure to properly orient and train the young worker who was injured. Beyond that, however, was the failure of the corporation to properly assess the hazard and because of that failure, to provide for it. This was, as I pointed out in my judgment, primarily a failure of the senior management and safety personnel but also in the supervision of the worker in question. [28]

In another case, the exploitation of young workers is highlighted:

At paragraphs 11 and 12, it is cited:

11.   In counsel's submission, the interests of the Union went beyond its institutional interest in being certified to represent employees of KES. In his submission, the facts of this case reveal an all too common situation where young workers are exploited in the workplace. They are taught certain tasks within the electrical trade, but are not provided with adequate training and supervision for the tasks of the entire trade. As such, they do not have any significant portability of their skills and are forced to continue to work for KES at sub-standard wages. [29]

12.   In addition, the applicant asserts that this situation is dangerous and leads to workplace injuries. It points out that in 2003 there were 30 workplace deaths in Ontario, 10 of which were suffered by persons under the age of 25. [30]

As noted in this next tragic case, untrained young workers can be deadly:

[35]   The employer hired two young workers (both in their 20s) from another company which was considered to be a leading company in the field of snubbing. The principal of the employer had previously worked for that other company as well, but he did not have knowledge or experience in snubbing. [31]

[38]   On February 4, 2004, the two young operators were working together, under the supervision of the site supervisor. The evidence indicates that following pressure testing of the gas line, the tubing hanger or dog nut was being removed from the stack. This requires that the tubing hanger be raised to a point in the stack where the diameter is bigger than the tubing hanger, so that the pressurized gas below can rush upward past the tubing hanger and be released through a valve. The tube is solid steel, so that the movement of the tubing hanger cannot be observed. [32]

[40]   However, the tubing hanger had not in fact been raised sufficiently, and it formed a seal preventing the upward movement of the pressurized gas below. The pressure above the tubing hanger had been released. The two young workers heard a

groaning sound from the pipe holding down the tubing hanger, due to the upward pressure being exerted on the tubing hanger from below.[33]

[42]   Upon realizing there was a problem, the snubbing operator ran up to the platform to join the junior snubbing operator. He did not refer to the pressure gauges, which would have shown the nature of the problem. Instead he opened the annular preventer to determine the cause of the problem. This had the effect of removing the last safety baffle preventing the tubing hanger from shooting up the stack.[34]

[43]   The review officer further noted:

The pipe remained, but it was groaning and twisting with the intense upward thrust. Now the only thing preventing a collapse of the pipe was the series of traveling slips which reinforced it. Despite the support of these "pinchers", however, the pipe was starting to bend with the pressure.

[The snubbing operator] then made a decision for which there is no satisfactory explanation. When he was interviewed, he explained that he next released the traveling slips in the hope that this might allow the pipe to straighten itself out. However, this action had the opposite result. With the last support on the pipe removed, the intense pressure from below caused it to bend and crumple, and the tubing hanger was suddenly propelled upward through the stack. Since the annular preventer had been opened, nothing stopped it from flying straight up the stack, with an explosive release of high pressure gas behind it. Unfortunately, this gas blasted out of a hole in the stack exactly where [the assistant snubbing operator] was standing....[35]

[44]   The assistant snubbing operator died when he was struck by pressurized gas as it was released in an uncontrolled manner.[36]

[50]   The October 31, 2008 decision by the review officer noted that the father of the deceased worker attended the oral hearing, and made an impassioned submission to the effect that the employer was grossly negligent in allowing two young men, with little practical experience, to operate a snubbing machine in this fashion without adequate supervision or safety procedures.[37]

These cases emphasize the need for OH&S officers to divide your recommendations into:

"1. Immediate or short-term corrective actions to eliminate or reduce the hazardous conditions and/or unsafe behaviors related to the accident."

2. Long-term system improvements to create or revise existing safety policies, programs plans, processes, procedures and practices identified as missing or inadequate in the investigation."[38]

Footnotes

1. *702 Accident Investigation*
Steven J. Geigle, MA, CET, CSHM
OSHAcademy Safety and Health Training
www.oshatrain.org

2 - 4. *Expert Advisory Panel on Occupational Health and Safety*
Report and Recommendations to the Minister of Labour
Issued: December 16, 2010
http://www.labour.gov.on.ca/english/hs/eap/report/index.php

4. Reference to 8.04 OCCUPATIONAL HEALTH AND SAFETY COMMITTEE
(Previously Article 20) cited in *Sensenbrenner Hospital v Canadian Office and
Professional Employees' Union, Local 523, 2012 CanLII 1799 (ON LA)*
Date: 2012-01-23
http://www.canlii.org/eliisa/highlight.do?text=OCCUPATIONAL+HEALTH+%26+SAF
ETY+a+good+recommendation&language=en&searchTitle=Search+all+CanLII+Databas
es&path=/en/on/onla/doc/2012/2012canlii1799/2012canlii1799.html

5 - 9. *20095291 (Re), 2009 CanLII 37310 (NB WHSCC)*
Date: 2009-06-08
Docket: 20095291
http://www.canlii.org/eliisa/highlight.do?text=OCCUPATIONAL+HEALTH+%26+SAF
ETY+a+good+recommendation&language=en&searchTitle=Search+all+CanLII+Databas
es&path=/en/nb/nbwhscc/doc/2009/2009canlii37310/2009canlii37310.html

10. *Joint Health and Safety Committees*
Revised May 2009
https://docs.google.com/viewer?a=v&q=cache:GLZNiJWE3f4J:www.worksafenb.ca/doc
s/JHS_Booklet_Eng.pdf+OH%26S+better+trained+committee+members+tend+to+have+
good+safety+records&hl=en&gl=uk&pid=bl&srcid=ADGEESiwUmlOaC9ES3EHywM
QEGyXp-
dkA4QPWAjWkBZMwkSWDkiwstV8OpHeOr5tklwXXS_7MYLa9XaimSYnveo4eTK7
uWP6AG8InegJnv9s_PkCBFicnfU2Vzk1lbMCJAjPu4nCcXvo&sig=AHIEtbR2jo8SiZcI
6NjOLEgFtJHnfWBprQ

11 - 17. *Canada: Joint Committees on Occupational Health and Safety*
Elaine Bernard
http://scholar.googleusercontent.com/scholar?q=cache:8CtnebQiQWEJ:scholar.google.co
m/+OH%26S+better+trained+committee+members+tend+to+have+good+safety+records
&hl=en&as_sdt=0,5

18 – 20. *Joint OH&S Committees*
https://www.bcnu.org/HealthSafety/HealthSafety.aspx?page=Joint%20OH&S%20Comm ittees

21 - 25. *Young People and Occupational Health and Safety: First Panel: Young People Speak*
2nd AWCBC Public Forum
Author: Kenneth George, Direction des relations avec les partenaires
https://docs.google.com/viewer?a=v&q=cache:eIjnSRvvms8J:www.awcbc.org/common/assets/english%2520pdf/textsession1aa.pdf+Workers+are+knowledgeable+about+the+OH%26S+concerns+in+their+workplaces+and+how+to+fix+them&hl=en&gl=ca&pid=bl&srcid=ADGEEShKu4TbC9U_IMM89uwAQ5SN4lPOOy8YykeW3tDMY3dngqf5B-GpJeWGp8sazw3-Os0RL_bCggB4_upcY8Ws15QexjRGd1hb7_PdXSCO437_ZEjaKaTGOcWXH2znP8n75obnXXr&sig=AHIEtbT8B_DF2JcGQHjW3ZdiKGXU-Vv9Sg

26 - 28. *R. v. Blue Ridge Lumber Inc., 2008 ABPC 310 (CanLII)*
Date: 2008-11-12
Docket: 041455783P1
http://www.canlii.org/eliisa/highlight.do?text=no+OCCUPATIONAL+HEALTH+%26+SAFETY+training+young+workers&language=en&searchTitle=Search+all+CanLII+Databases&path=/en/ab/abpc/doc/2008/2008abpc310/2008abpc310.html

29 - 30. *International Brotherhood of Electrical Workers, Local 586 v. KE Electrical Services Ltd., 2005 CanLII 35125 (ON LRB)*
Date: 2005-09-26
Docket: 0188-05-HS
http://www.canlii.org/eliisa/highlight.do?text=no+OCCUPATIONAL+HEALTH+%26+SAFETY+training+young+workers&language=en&searchTitle=Search+all+CanLII+Databases&path=/en/on/onlrb/doc/2005/2005canlii35125/2005canlii35125.html

31 – 37. *WCAT-2010-00104 (Re), 2010 CanLII 23340 (BC WCAT)*
Date: 2010-01-13
Docket: WCAT-2010-00104
http://www.canlii.org/eliisa/highlight.do?text=no+OCCUPATIONAL+HEALTH+%26+SAFETY+training+young+workers&language=en&searchTitle=Search+all+CanLII+Databases&path=/en/bc/bcwcat/doc/2010/2010canlii23340/2010canlii23340.html

38. *702 Accident Investigation*
Steven J. Geigle, MA, CET, CSHM
OSHAcademy Safety and Health Training
www.oshatrain.org

Appendix 3

Recommendations to Improve Workplace Health and Safety in Ontario
http://www.kmblaw.com/news83.html

In January 2010, the Minister of Labour, the Honourable Peter Fonseca, appointed an Expert Advisory Panel to conduct a comprehensive review of Ontario's Occupational Health and Safety Prevention and Enforcement system with the goal of improving workplace health and safety in the province.

On December 16, 2010, the 10-member panel, which included members from the labour, employer and academic communities with workplace health and safety expertise, submitted its recommendations to the Minister. The panel made a total of 46 recommendations.

Key Recommendations:

■*Creation of a new prevention organization within the Ministry of Labour, chaired by a Chief Prevention Officer, which will be tasked with coordinating and aligning prevention system strategies, priorities and programs, and overseeing Ontario's Health and Safety Associations.*

■*Currently, the prevention function is the responsibility of the Workplace Safety and Insurance Board.*

■*Mandatory training of Health and Safety Representatives and health and safety awareness training for all workers and supervisors prior to being exposed to workplace hazards.*

■*Training program would include the rights and responsibilities of workers and supervisors, the roles of workplace parties and the definition of a hazard.*

■*Mandatory entry-level training for construction workers.*

■*Mandatory training for high-hazard work, including fall-protection training for workers working at heights.*

■*Tougher penalties for deliberate or repeat offences that immediately place workers at risk.*

■*Improve the protection for new workers, youth and recent immigrants through mandatory training, creation of safety-related materials in multiple languages, and the establishment of a committee to provide advice on issues related to vulnerable workers.*

■*The Ministry of Labour and Ontario Labour Relations Board should work together to develop a process to expedite the resolution of reprisal complaints under Section 50 of the Occupational Health and Safety Act ("OHSA").*

■*Section 50 is intended to enable workers to raise health and safety concerns and exercise their rights under the OHSA, including refusing unsafe work without fear of employers dismissing or otherwise penalizing workers for exercising such rights.*

■*Better support for small businesses.*

■*Creation of a small business committee to advise the Minister on the needs of owners and workers in small business.*

■*Intensify support for small business compliance through the creation of focused and integrated programs dedicated to enforcement and prevention activities for the small business sector.*

■*Improved occupational health and safety training in primary and secondary schools, colleges and universities.*

The Panel's Report highlights the need for enhanced training for all workers and health and safety representatives, greater access to occupational health and safety resources and support, the need for more prevention programs, and greater support for workers and owners in the small business sector.

The Honourable Premier Dalton McGuinty has welcomed the recommendations and immediately announced the creation of a Chief Prevention Officer position to ensure effective health and safety services and enforcement at workplaces.

The recommendation of providing better support for the small business sector is a welcomed initiative as these employers lack sufficient human resources support to adequately meet their requirements under the OHSA and ensure worker safety. Unfortunately, all employers must be wary of the Panel's recommendation for increased penalties for non-compliance.

To view the Panel's Report in its entirety, please click on the following link:
http://www.labour.gov.on.ca/english/hs/eap/report/index.php

If you would like to discuss your obligations under the OHSA, please do not hesitate to contact any one of the following lawyers who practice in the Occupational Health and Safety Field in our Labour and Employment Law Group:

Chapter 10 – "Hazard Analysis"

As out course emphasized:

*"*The goal of the hazard identification and control program is to make the workplace and its operations as safe as possible and to keep employees from being harmed. It is an ongoing program that is actually never finished."[1]

As noted, identifying hazards can be by area:

"Static worksites such as factories are well suited to a hazard identification method involving grouping hazards into common types and identifying them by surveying all the different areas of the site"[2] [see Appendix 4 cited below].

As reported, these can include:

"1. Get an up-to-date plan of the worksite. This must provide an accurate picture of the work area.

2. Get a chart that shows the process of production or work flow. If one doesn't exist, then compile such a chart.

3. Divide the worksite into identifiable areas and number them. This division can be based on how the production is carried out or the physical layout of a site.

For example, a small factory may contain: Stores area — Production area — Workshops — Offices — Yards

4. Ask staff in all areas to list what they consider are potential hazards in the places they work and why they consider that they are hazards/potential hazards. Also get them to make a list of the chemicals/substances they use.

Use a data collection form like that given in appendix B to gather the information. Be sure to attach the hazard information sheets to the form, so people know what type of hazards they are looking for."[3]

One can also analyze hazards by examining the work to be done:

"Work that is not done on a static site is probably better analysed by first identifying the different occupations involved and the work people carry out, then the hazards they face doing that work."[4]

As cited, this can include:

"1. Identify all the tasks people carry out. A task consists of a number of steps, actions or stages performed in order to complete a specific work assignment.

2. Work out the steps or stages involved in doing the task — using the sheet provided in appendix C or one you have drawn up yourself, and getting those involved to help.

3. Using the list of hazards in Appendix 4 [cited below], *ask those involved what they consider apply to each step identified and to write them down.*

4. Use existing resources such as guidelines, codes of practice, information booklets, manufacturers' information, reports from inspectors/consultants, complaints, environmental monitoring reports; and

Especially use records of accidents, illnesses and near-misses — not only from within your company, but also within your industry — to ensure all hazards are identified.

5. Use the information derived from task analysis to build up a profile of hazards and the occupations and tasks they apply to. This can be done on a computer database using key words so hazards common to a wide range of occupations can be identified. "[5]

Finally, as named, "a more technical approach to hazard identification is to identify the processes involved on a worksite and go through each process step-by-step, identifying the hazards at each step of the process."[6]

This can include:

"1. Make an inventory of all substances/chemicals used in the process.

2. List the process from where the material is delivered to the factory / site to where the finished goods are dispatched. Identifying the steps where material is transformed by physical and chemical means.

3. Draw up a flow chart detailing every step of the process and detailing the various stages where chemicals and substances are used in the process.

4. Identify all the hazards at each stage of the process.

5. Use existing resources, such as regulations, codes of practice, information booklets, manufacturers' information, reports from inspectors/consultants, complaints, environmental monitoring reports; and

Especially use records of accidents, illnesses and near-misses, not only within your company but within your industry, to ensure all hazards are identified.

6. Summarise the information collected. "[7]

As the following case[8] emphasizes, a work place can be anything, including a crane, and as such needs a hazard assessment in its own right.

"The crane being used for this operation was a Linkbelt Conventional Crawler Crane, model 1.S108B, Serial Number 9LG3041, Unit C1000 equipped with a 60.96 centimetre pile driver (hereinafter "the Crane"). The Crane constitutes a "Worksite" within the meaning of the Occupational Health and Safety Act."[9]

"The key element of culpability in this case is the failure of Agra Foundations Limited to conduct a hazard assessment on the crane prior to commencing work at the Expocrete site. The Defence admits that it failed to conduct the necessary hazard assessment and it admits that the crane was a work site as defined under the Occupational Health and Safety Act, RSA 2000, Chapter 0-2, as amended."[10]

And:

"Although Agra had a number of policies and procedures that had been given to employees regarding work processes on cranes, a hazard assessment on the Crane had not been conducted prior to commencing work at the Expocrete site."[11]

As further emphasized, had a hazard assessment been conducted it would have identified:

> *"a.   that the master clutch on the Crane was reversed resulting in the need for the operator to take extra care to ensure the draw works were disengaged when they were supposed to be; and*
>
> *b.   that the practice of opening the doors to the draw works to cool the machinery down would necessitate extra caution when working around that area of the Crane."*[12]

Even with apparent adequate procedures in place, hazards can escape notice as cited at paragraphs 15 and 18 in this case:

"[15]   Under the internal responsibility system at Dana Canada, everyone was responsible for safety in the workplace and workers were encouraged to identify safety hazards and report them to their supervisors for corrective action. The Thorold Frame Plant had its own Human Resources Department with a manager responsible for health and safety. There was also a functioning Joint Health and Safety Committee made up of three company representatives and three union representatives that met monthly to inspect the facilities and identify safety hazards. They had not identified the calibration process as a safety hazard."[13]

[18]   Dana Canada has had a risk management team in place since the fall of 2005. Since then they have developed over 50 health and safety directives and guidelines

for their plants in Canada. They also have an annual assessment and auditing process utilizing third party auditors to ensure compliance with these directives and guidelines as well as legislated health and safety guidelines. In Ontario, Dana spends in excess of $250,000 annually on third party consultants and a further $400,000 annually on staff salaries, safety supplies and internal training to maintain and improve its existing safety programs.[14]

And missing a hazard can be costly as noted at paragraphs 19 and 20:

"[19]   While I am impressed by the steps that Dana Canada has taken over the past few years, general deterrence remains the paramount factor to be considered here. The costs incurred by Dana Canada in taking these steps illustrate how expensive it can be for a company to comply with safety laws. I must keep that in mind and ensure that the fine I impose is not seen as a licence fee for those who do not comply with those laws.

[20]   Accordingly, I am imposing a fine of $80,000."[15]

In terms of hazards, it was emphasized that it is impossible to eliminate all hazards and to form legislation to do so would require the unrealistic elimination of most, if not all, employment:

517 - This requirement is inherently confusing and unrealistic. It could be read to require the Secretary to ban all occupations in which there remains some risk of injury, impaired health, or life expectancy. In the case of all occupations, it will be impossible to eliminate all risks to safety and health. Thus, the present criteria could, if literally applied, close every business in this nation. In addition, in many cases, the standard which might most `adequately' and `feasibly' assure the elimination of the danger would be the prohibition of the occupation itself." Leg. Hist. 367 (comments of Sen. Dominick on his proposed amendment No. 1054) (emphasis in original).[16]

518 - In the ensuing floor debate on this issue, Senator Dominick reiterated his concern that "[i]t is unrealistic to attempt. as [the Committee's § 6 (b) (5)] apparently does, to establish a utopia free from any hazards. Absolute safety is an impossibility . . . ." 116 Cong. Rec. 37614 (1970), Leg. Hist. 480.[35] The Senator concluded: "Any administrator responsible 518*518 for enforcing the statute will be faced with an impossible choice. Either he must forbid employment in all occupations where there is any risk of injury, even if the technical state of the art could not remove the hazard, or he must ignore the mandate of Congress . . . ." 116 Cong. Rec., at 37614, Leg. Hist. 481-482.[17]

Nevertheless, investigations of hazards can include warrantless searches as needed.

As cited:

596 - In this case we consider whether § 103 (a) of the Federal Mine Safety and Health Act of 1977, 30 U. S. C. § 813 (a) (1976 ed., Supp. III), which authorizes warrantless inspections of underground and surface mines, violates the Fourth Amendment. Concluding that searches conducted pursuant to this provision are reasonable within the meaning of the Fourth Amendment, we reverse the judgment of the District Court for the Eastern District of Wisconsin invalidating the statute.[18]

597 - The Federal Mine Safety and Health Act of 1977, 91 Stat. 1290, 30 U. S. C. § 801 et seq. (1976 ed. and Supp. III), requires the Secretary of Labor to develop detailed mandatory health and safety standards to govern the operation of the Nation's mines. 30 U. S. C. § 811 (1976 ed., Supp. III).[1] Section 103 (a) of the Act, 30 U. S. C. § 813 (a) (1976 ed., Supp. III), provides that federal mine inspectors are to inspect underground mines at least four times per year and surface mines at least twice a year to insure compliance with these standards, and to make followup inspections to determine whether previously discovered violations have been corrected. This section also grants mine inspectors "a right of entry to, upon, or through any coal or other mine"[2] and states that "no advance notice of an inspection shall be provided to any person." If a mine operator refuses to allow a warrantless inspection conducted pursuant to § 103 (a), the Secretary 597*597 is authorized to institute a civil action to obtain injunctive or other appropriate relief. 30 U. S. C. § 818 (a) (1) (C) (1976 ed., Supp. III).[19]

In this other case, there was a warrantless search violation although the results may surprise the reader:

As cited at paragraphs 1 and 2:

"[1]   On March 8, 2000, a brickworker, Frank Aquino was crushed by a dehacker machine at the Burlington plant of Canada Brick (the company). He survived his injuries but never worked again."[20]

"[2]   As a result of the industrial accident, Canada Brick was charged under a provincial regulatory statute:

Canada Brick Limited/Briques Canada Limitee, 5155 Dundas Street West, Burlington, Ontario L7R 3X4 about the 8th day of March, 2000, at the City of Burlington, in the Central West Region in the Province of Ontario did commit the offence of failing, as an employer, to take every precaution reasonable in the circumstances for the protection of a worker at a workplace, located at Dundas Street West, Burlington, contrary to section 25(2)(h) of the Occupational Health and Safety Act, R.S.O. 1990, c.O.1."[21]

As further stated at paragraph 157(10):

(10)   The bright line rule for the division of inspection and investigatory functions, in terms of the scope of s.8 Charter protection, occurs when "an adversarial relationship crystallizes" between the subject of government scrutiny and the government official(s).

Although the government and the company under inspection may, during an inspection, be in "opposing positions", when the government "exercises its investigative function [it is]...in a more traditional adversarial relationship" attracting the more robust protection of section 8 of the Charter: R. v. Jarvis, at p.37. Accordingly, in the circumstances of any particular case, the adversarial relationship crystallizes "when the predominant purpose of an official's inquiry is the determination of penal liability" where "a liberty interest is at stake": R. v. Jarvis, at pp.9, 24, 37, 39; R. v. Ling, at p.50.[22]

Where the court states the assessment has to be on an individual basis, at 157(11):

(11)   The application of the "predominant purpose" test involves a case-by-case examination of the conduct of the government official(s) in the totality of the circumstances – "There is no clear formula" otherwise: R. v. Jarvis, at p.39. All factors that bear upon the nature of the government inquiry must be considered. While the existence of reasonable grounds to believe an offence may have occurred is not in and of itself a sufficient indicator that the state is conducting a de facto investigation, "In most cases, if all ingredients of an offence are reasonably thought to have occurred, it is likely that the investigation function is triggered": R. v. Jarvis, at p.39. Although it cannot be said that "from the moment such suspicion is formed, an investigation has begun" (R. v. Jarvis, at p.40), there may, in a given case, come a point where continuation of warrantless inquiry becomes constitutionally unreasonable – in effect, "the same conduct motivated by a different purpose may interfere with reasonable expectations of privacy": R. v. D'Amour, at p.496.[23]

With a differentiation described at 157(12):

(12)   The reason regulatory inspectors have been granted powers of inspection is to determine whether an offence has been committed requiring an immediate or near-immediate response in furtherance of public safety – "the very nature of an administrative inspection in a regulated industry [is] that it takes place when there are no reasonable grounds to believe that a particular offence has been committed" (emphasis of original): Comité Paritaire v. Potash, at pp.452-3. "There is an important distinction between having reasonable and probable grounds to believe that an offence was committed and simply having information": Comité Paritaire v. Potash, at p.454. On occasion, during an inspection, government discovery of non-compliance with regulatory standards warrants an instant remedial response under government direction or order. Prolonged attendance, inquiries, inspections, questioning and even seizures by government officials may prove necessary to effect abatement and timely compliance in the interests of public welfare and protection. In these circumstances, the exercise of warrantless powers does not offend our constitutional notion of reasonableness. What is offensive, however, is over-holding in the use of such powers into a disguised investigation or "Quite conceivably, situations may arise in which charges are delayed" improperly in order to compel the target to provide evidence against itself: R. v. Jarvis, at p.40; R. v. Chusid 2001 CanLII 28348 (ON SC), (2002), 57 O.R. (3d) 20 (S.C.J.), at pp.39-41.[24]

The OH&S warrantless search was proper, as cited at paragraph 158:

[158]   The trial court correctly accepted that Insp. Burke's attendance at the Canada Brick premises on March 8, 2000 in response to notification of the Ministry of Labour concerning the Aquino accident was an inspection authorized by law. The government, in furtherance of its statutory mandate to monitor safe workplaces, was obliged to straightaway determine the circumstances of the reported industrial accident in order to ascertain whether it was the result of non-compliance with the Act or Regulations and if so, to take the necessary and timely steps to protect other workers from a similar mishap. To this end, on March 8, 2000, Insp. Burke properly exercised the panoply of warrantless powers conferred by s.54(1) of the O.H.S.A. in an effort to learn how the accident occurred, whether it was the product of a preventable hazard, and what remedial action, if any, was required.[25]

Resulting in a stop-work order:

[159]   In a matter of a couple of hours, Insp. Burke concluded that the unguarded walkway in the path of the moving head of the dehacker machine amounted to an unreasonably dangerous location for workers. He issued a stop work order being of the view, pursuant to ss.57(1)(6) of the Act, that a contravention of the Act or Regulations existed constituting "a danger or hazard to the health or safety" of workers.[26]

However, it was determined that during the above mentioned process:

[160]   ... Insp. Burke had become aware of the non-compliance with the Parco order made almost seven months earlier. In these circumstances, certainly from an objective point of view, Insp. Burke had reasonable grounds for believing Canada Brick had contravened s.25(2)(h) of the Act.[27]

As the court emphasized:

[162]   The legitimate use of warrantless, administrative authority expired on or about March 8, 2000. [28]

Whereas, the continuing investigation of this other apparent infraction [*Parco*] and the collection of evidence was not protected:

"The predominate objective of Insp. Burke thereafter was the investigative gathering of evidence respecting liability for the regulatory infraction whether or not he would ultimately see himself as having grounds to charge the company."[29]

"This became a warrantless search no longer authorized by law."[30]

"Deliberate deferral of consideration as to whether he had reasonable grounds or whether such grounds objectively existed does not alter the transparently clear dominant intent of the inspector in the three weeks following March 8."[31]

"No longer exercising statutory powers toward remediation of a workplace hazard, the inspector's investigation improperly secured evidence without valid consent or any warrant to search."[32]

As such:

[164]   Canada Brick's s.8 Charter right was breached by the government's prolonged employ of administrative powers to gather evidence as to whether an offence had been committed.[33]

However, the court ruled:

[171]   Insp. Burke's unconstitutional search must be understood contextually.

Although he improperly exercised warrantless search powers to further investigative efforts, there is no real support in the trial record, nor persuasive suggestion in argument on this appeal, that the state agent acted as he did knowing that he ought to have secured warrant authority.

It is apparent that Insp. Burke believed he was legally justified in investigating through the use of warrantless powers conferred by the O.H.S.A. and deferring any consideration of the relevance of the objective existence of reasonable grounds until his evidence was gathered ...

The integrity of the administration of justice has not been unduly threatened.

The government's actions would not shock the conscience of the community.

In these circumstances, there is no established pattern of abuse or threat of future departure from constitutional compliance with s.8 Charter standards.[34]

Others have also summarized the salient points:

"The Ontario Superior Court of Justice has once again considered the difficult issue of where the line should be drawn between inspections by government regulators and investigations that seek to gather evidence with a view to laying charges."[35]

"The former, if authorized by statute, can be carried out without a formal search warrant but the latter cannot without violating section 8 of the Canadian Charter of Rights and Freedoms, the provision that guarantees the right to be free from unreasonable search and seizure."[36]

In R. v. Canada Brick Ltd. (June 30, 2005), "the legitimate use of warrantless, administrative authority expired on or about March 8, 2000."[37]

"The predominant objective of [the inspector] thereafter was the investigative gathering of evidence respecting liability for the regulatory infraction whether or not he would ultimately see himself as having grounds to charge the company."[38]

"This became a warrantless search no longer authorized by law."[39]

"However, despite this ruling, the Court declined to issue a stay of proceedings, noting that there was no evidence that the inspector had known that he should have secured a search warrant."[40]

"The Court expressed the view that the integrity of the administration of justice had not been threatened by the government's conduct and that there was no established pattern of abuse or threat of future non-compliance with Charter standards."[41]

As such:

"The point at which a warrantless inspection becomes an investigation requiring a search warrant is when an adversarial relationship crystallizes between the subject of the investigation and the investigator."[42]

"That point is reached when 'the predominant purpose' of the inspector's inquiry is the determination of liability when there is a liberty interest at stake for the subject of the investigation."[43]

"The Court was clear that the mere making of a stop work order under section 57 of the OHSA does not serve to crystallize that adversarial relationship."[44]

"This is so despite the fact that a stop work order is premised on the inspector finding that a provision of the Act or regulations has been contravened."[45]

"The Court held that, the finding of a contravention alone does not mean that the inspector knows who is responsible for the contravention or how the unsafe work conditions came about."[46]

Footnotes

1. *704 Hazard Analysis*
Steven J. Geigle, MA, CET, CSHM
OSHAcademy Safety and Health Training
http://www.oshatrain.org/courses/mods/704e.html

2 - 7. *How to Identify and Control Hazards: A workbook*
Published by the Occupational Safety and Health Service of the Department of Labour
December 1992
Revised January 1994
https://docs.google.com/viewer?a=v&q=cache:u7EQmlQKWyoJ:www.osh.govt.nz/order
/catalogue/archive/identifyhazards.pdf+identifying,+analyzing+and+controlling+hazards
+in+the+workplace&hl=en&gl=uk&pid=bl&srcid=ADGEESiM30zlGIRVvHTRHupcv2
HZLTdqDQ1O1S7mq4qNMaSTvCc4XB8Tccv-e62oxdgJ6H_zwFYOVzzpw6waR-
ZIq_uTNUUi4QXvDv4OFjHgL30aHcMHOy6uXhUcw-
32Tq5fxGm_hzjV&sig=AHIEtbQS7ikApTYoanSWqadSmByEnzQJ0Q

8 - 12. *R. v. Agra Foundations Limited, 2011 ABPC 224 (CanLII)*
Date: 2011-07-19
Docket: 090867185P10101-0102
http://www.canlii.org/eliisa/highlight.do?text=OCCUPATIONAL+HEALTH+%26+SAF
ETY+hazards+not+identified&language=en&searchTitle=Search+all+CanLII+Databa
ses&path=/en/ab/abpc/doc/2011/2011abpc224/2011abpc224.html

13 - 15. *Ontario (Ministry of Labour) v. Dana Canada Corporation, 2009 ONCJ 11 (CanLII)*
Date: 2009-01-06
Docket: 2111-998-06-3983
http://www.canlii.org/eliisa/highlight.do?text=OCCUPATIONAL+HEALTH+%26+SAF
ETY+hazards+not+identified&language=en&searchTitle=Search+all+CanLII+Databases
&path=/en/on/oncj/doc/2009/2009oncj11/2009oncj11.html

16 - 17. *AMERICAN TEXTILE MANUFACTURERS INSTITUTE, INC., ET AL. v. DONOVAN, SECRETARY OF LABOR, ET AL.*
452 U.S. 490 (1981)
No. 79-1429.
Supreme Court of United States.
Argued January 21, 1981.
Decided June 17, 1981.
http://scholar.google.co.uk/scholar_case?case=16807219216043765696&q=OCCUPATI
ONAL+HEALTH+%26+SAFETY+hazards+not+identified&hl=en&as_sdt=2,5

18 - 19. *DONOVAN, SECRETARY OF LABOR v. DEWEY ET AL.*
452 U.S. 594 (1981)
No. 80-901.
Supreme Court of United States.
Argued April 28, 1981.
Decided June 17, 1981.
http://scholar.google.co.uk/scholar_case?case=13160281078217041331&q=OCCUPATI
ONAL+HEALTH+%26+SAFETY+hazards+not+identified&hl=en&as_sdt=2,5

20 - 34. *R. v. Canada Brick Ltd., 2005 CanLII 24925 (ON SC)*
Date: 2005-06-30
Docket: M2266/03
http://www.canlii.org/eliisa/highlight.do?text=R.+v.+Canada+Brick+Ltd.+%28June+30
%2C+2005%29&language=en&searchTitle=Search+all+CanLII+Databases&path=/en/on
/onsc/doc/2005/2005canlii24925/2005canlii24925.html

35 - 46. *Ontario Court holds that health and safety inspector violated Charter guarantee
against unreasonable search and seizure*
http://www.ehlaw.ca/publications/dec05/CanadaBrickLtd.shtml

Appendix 4

Reference to Appendix A cited in How to Identify and Control Hazards: A workbook
Published by the Occupational Safety and Health Service of the Department of Labour
December 1992
Revised January 1994
https://docs.google.com/viewer?a=v&q=cache:u7EQmlQKWyoJ:www.osh.govt.nz/order
/catalogue/archive/identifyhazards.pdf+identifying,+analyzing+and+controlling+hazards
+in+the+workplace&hl=en&gl=uk&pid=bl&srcid=ADGEESiM30zlGIRVvHTRHupcv2
HZLTdqDQ1O1S7mq4qNMaSTvCc4XB8Tccv-e62oxdgJ6H_zwFYOVzzpw6waR-
ZIq_uTNUUi4QXvDv4OFjHgL30aHcMHOy6uXhUcw-
32Tq5fxGm_hzjV&sig=AHIEtbQS7ikApTYoanSWqadSmByEnzQJ0Q

CHEMICAL HAZARDS

*Chemicals can affect the skin by contact or they affect the body either through the
digestive system or via the lungs if air is contaminated with chemicals, vapour, mist or
dust.*

*There can be an acute effect, i.e. the person is affected immediately, or there can be a
chronic effect, i.e. the person is affected in the medium to long term due to the
accumulation of chemical or substances in or on the body.*

NOISE HAZARDS

*Excessive noise can disrupt concentration, interfere with communication, and result in
loss of hearing. High impact noises are particularly damaging. Noise can also mask out
signals, affecting communication.*

RADIATION HAZARDS

*Ionising radiation is in such equipment as radioactive gauging devices or the radioactive
trace element used in analytical chemistry. Non-ionising radiation covers infrared
radiation (heat-producing processes), lasers, ultraviolet radiation (welding, sunlight),
and microwaves (high-frequency welders, freeze drying).*

ELECTRICAL HAZARDS

This covers the risk of injury from all forms of electrical energy.

LIGHTING HAZARDS

*Inadequate lighting levels are a potential safety hazard. A common problem area is the
reaction time needed for the eyes to adjust from a brightly lit to a darker environment —*

such as forklift driver coming indoors from bright sunlight. Temporary lighting is often inadequate.

VIBRATION HAZARDS

This includes whole-body vibration — e.g. truck drivers, people standing on vibrating platforms, and operators of mobile equipment — and also segmental vibration effects from such equipment as hand tools, chainsaws, and pneumatic hammers.

TEMPERATURE HAZARDS

Extremes of cold or heat can cause problems due to individual fatigue or reduced capacity to work.

BIOLOGICAL HAZARDS

These include insects, bacteria, fungi, plants, worms, animals and viruses. For example, poultry workers exposed to bird feathers and droppings to which they are allergic can contract a medical condition. Brucellosis is a well known problem in New Zealand associated with people handling meat and meat products infected with brucella. Hepatitis and the AIDS virus are other biological hazards.

ERGONOMIC HAZARDS

This covers risk of injury from manual handling procedures, incorrectly designed work stations, audio and visual alarms, and colour coding control mechanisms.

PHYSICAL HAZARDS

This includes a wide range of risks of injury — as diverse as being caught in or by machinery, buried in trenches or hurt by collapsing machinery. This category also includes the hazards from working in confined spaces, being hit by flying objects, caught in explosions, falling from heights and tripping on obstacles.

MISCELLANEOUS HAZARDS

This includes stress, fatigue, the effects of shiftwork, and even assaults from other people.

Chapter 11 – Radiation Hazards

This book has given a flavor to occupational hazards, some legislation related to such accidents, and now with the dwindling stocks of oil[1] and possible increase in nuclear powered generation stations, let's look at this hazard.

As further cited previously, in terms of hazards, it was emphasized that it is impossible to eliminate all hazards and to form legislation to do so would require the unrealistic elimination of most, if not all, employment:

517 - This requirement is inherently confusing and unrealistic. It could be read to require the Secretary to ban all occupations in which there remains some risk of injury, impaired health, or life expectancy. In the case of all occupations, it will be impossible to eliminate all risks to safety and health. Thus, the present criteria could, if literally applied, close every business in this nation. In addition, in many cases, the standard which might most `adequately' and `feasibly' assure the elimination of the danger would be the prohibition of the occupation itself." Leg. Hist. 367 (comments of Sen. Dominick on his proposed amendment No. 1054) (emphasis in original).[2]

518 - In the ensuing floor debate on this issue, Senator Dominick reiterated his concern that "[i]t is unrealistic to attempt. as [the Committee's § 6 (b) (5)] apparently does, to establish a utopia free from any hazards. Absolute safety is an impossibility . . . ." 116 Cong. Rec. 37614 (1970), Leg. Hist. 480.[35] The Senator concluded: "Any administrator responsible 518*518 for enforcing the statute will be faced with an impossible choice. Either he must forbid employment in all occupations where there is any risk of injury, even if the technical state of the art could not remove the hazard, or he must ignore the mandate of Congress . . . ." 116 Cong. Rec., at 37614, Leg. Hist. 481-482.[3]

Hazards of radiation accidents are someone expected by "the nature of the beast", but to legislate against such events would be practically impossible:

Winnipeg Free Press

December 27, 2012   NO CLASSES TODAY

Manitoba's forgotten nuclear accident
By: Dave Taylor
Posted: 03/24/2011
http://www.winnipegfreepress.com/opinion/westview/manitobas-forgotten-nuclear-accident-118563039.html

The nuclear disaster unfolding in Japan has provoked horror and sadness around the world, but also relief in those who believe they will never be vulnerable to such a disaster. Manitoba, of course, will never need to fear a Japanese-scale catastrophe, but unknown to most people, it did experience its own severe nuclear event in November 1978.

The WR-1 reactor at Pinawa, which was cooled by a type of oil (terphenyl isomer), experienced a major coolant leak as one of the pipes developed a hole and 2,739 litres of oil leaked.

It took several weeks for workers in protective gear to pinpoint and repair it, according to a Winnipeg Free Press article, (July 30, 1981). Much of the leaked oil was then discharged into the Winnipeg River. According to Dr. Agnes Bishop of the Atomic Energy Control Board, (now the CNSC), the fuel reached high temperatures.

Although the temperature did not hit the meltdown level, it did result in three fuel elements being broken with some fission products being released. The accident, which many would consider significant especially to the health and safety of Manitobans, took several years to be reported to the province.

An attempt was made in 2000 to have the report from this accident made public, but Atomic Energy of Canada refused, and labelled it "Protected."

We may never know what nasty radioactive carcinogens were vented or released into the air and water of our province.

Such is the nature of the beast. Exemptions under Canada's Freedom of Information Act significantly compromise the transparency of the industry in our country. Canada has entrusted its plan for nuclear waste disposal with the corporations who produce the waste, a clear conflict of interest

In fact, it apparently took a number of "environmental" radiation accidents to prompt America to tackle such events, legislatively.

"Unexpected events such as environmental catastrophes capture wide public attention. Soon after five major shocks—Three Mile Island, Love Canal, Bhopal, Chernobyl, and the Exxon Valdez oil spill—Congress voted on new risk regulation."[4]

However, as cited:

"Matthew Kahn links to a 2007 paper he wrote on this subject, which finds that, while oil-spill-type disasters do force new regulations onto the legislative agenda, they don't make lawmakers any more likely to vote for them."[5]

In fact:

"Conventional wisdom holds that environmental disasters lead Congress to toughen regulatory standards. But a new UCLA study has found that members of Congress were less likely to take pro-green positions on legislation in the wake of such disasters than at other times during the same calendar year."[6]

"The reason? Legislation following these environmental 'shocks' is typically written by those with strong pro-environment voting records who propose more radical legislation. Such legislation tends to overreach, leading moderates and more conservative lawmakers to vote against the bills."[7]

"Environmental disasters polarize the Congress; they're not uniting Congress," said Matthew E. Kahn, a professor at the UCLA Institute of the Environment and author of the study. "Environmental disasters give environmentalists the upper hand by changing the parameters of debate. In the aftermath of a shock such as the Exxon Valdez oil spill, the news media provide extensive coverage, members of Congress know that voters expect them to 'do something' and environmentalists are aware that they may be able to enact 'greener' legislation. The polluter faces a nasty public relations problem and must decide how to lobby the Congress and the people to minimize the extra regulation it faces due to the event.[8]

"The result," Kahn said, "is often legislation that goes too far and turns off those who had taken the pro-environment position on other legislation in the same year."[9]

Well, if legislative remedies won't work – what should nuclear power companies do?

According to Canada's prime minister, $650 million should do?

As cited:

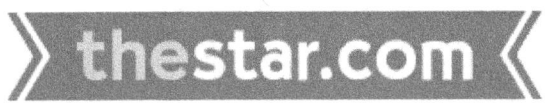

How much would a nuclear meltdown cost?
By Tyler Hamilton, Energy and Technology Columnist
Published on Monday November 30, 2009
http://www.thestar.com/business/article/732384--how-much-would-a-nuclear-meltdown-cost

What kind of insurance policy do you take out if you operate a large nuclear plant in one of the most densely populated, fastest-growing communities in Canada?

The Harper government believes $650 million should cover it off, even in the event of a catastrophic, however improbable, accident at a nuclear plant such as the aging Pickering generating station.

Whether that amount is high enough was the subject of lengthy debate these past two weeks as legislators took a close look at Bill C-20, the Nuclear Liability and Compensation Act.

The bill raises the cap on liability to $650 million from the $75 million limit established in 1976. It represents a nearly ninefold increase that the federal government calls "reasonable" and in line with international standards, given the extremely low likelihood of a severe accident. But critics of the bill say the government is still lowballing the cost of potential damages and is out of touch with other nuclear-power nations that measure liability in the billions, not millions of dollars.

"Under any scenario of a major nuclear accident happening within Canadian nuclear facilities, you can crack through $650 million without breaking a sweat," said B.C. MP Nathan Cullen, the New Democrat for Skeena-Bulkley Valley, who's on the parliamentary committee combing through the bill. The difference between a $650 million event and a multibillion-dollar catastrophe, he said, can be determined by the direction and speed of the wind that carries the radiation.

Cullen, speaking later in an interview, said it would be a mistake to dismiss these concerns as fear mongering. "Everybody seems to be so shy of mentioning those words, `nuclear accident.' But we have to imagine it, unfortunately."

He said citizens of Pickering and Toronto should be following the issue more closely, with four reactors at the Pickering B nuclear station soon to reach the end of their safe operating lives. Ontario Power Generation is to decide by year's end whether to refurbish the four to extend their operation to 2060.

Alternatively, OPG may seek a short-term life extension as part of a strategy for "maximizing asset value" – similar to the five-year life extension given to Atomic Energy of Canada's NRU isotope-producing reactor in Chalk River.

The NRU reactor was supposed to cease operating by the end of 2005 but its licence was extended to 2011. A heavy water leak forced the reactor to shut down in May 2009 for repairs. Six months later Atomic Energy scientists are still working on a fix.

In the United States, liability for nuclear accidents is set at $10 billion (U.S.), while in Japan the cap will be doubled next year to roughly $1.47 billion (Canadian). In Germany, there is no cap on nuclear liability but an operator must be able to cover at least $4 billion.

On an end note, this blog may be appropriate:

The nature of the beast we have come to call growth.[10]

"However, the real danger still exists, and that is our obsession for Growth. In general a country's energy appetite gets fatter and fatter in direct proportion to its economic growth. To keep up with the 'growth' ladder, human civilisation has moved from wood to coal, coal to oil, and ultimately oil to nukes. The age of easy oil is over. We have already burnt too much of fossil fuels (up to a point that it dug a hole in the ozone layer), the natural gas bases are shrinking as well."[11]

"Too many of us are consuming too many resources too fast in the name of economic growth. The expansion of the global nuclear industry (based on today's apparent affluence of Uranium) is therefore, the inevitable by-product of the hysterical expansion of the "growth" economy."[12]

"The Roman civilisation ran on slavery. The 21st century civilisation runs on energy."[13]

"And the universal energy law runs on a simple algebra: The more and more you dig, the less and less you get. The less and less you get, the more and more energy you require to dig deeper and deeper."[14]

"It comes to a point where digging deeper requires more energy than what it actually gets from digging. The end game is simple: sooner or later the global enterprise of 'digging & drilling' will be asking for a bail out."[15]

"Indeed, the earth's natural resources are finite. If we keep digging for them, we will eventually exhaust them."[16]

"It has become a matter of simple common sense."[17]

Footnotes

1. "Three Reasons for Investing Now in Fossil Fuel Conservation: Technological Lock-In, Institutional Inertia, and Oil Wars"
Richard W. England
Journal of Economic Issues, Vol. 28, No. 3 (Sep., 1994), pp. 755-776
 Published by: Association for Evolutionary Economics

2 - 3. *AMERICAN TEXTILE MANUFACTURERS INSTITUTE, INC., ET AL. v. DONOVAN, SECRETARY OF LABOR, ET AL.*
452 U.S. 490 (1981)
No. 79-1429.
Supreme Court of United States.
Argued January 21, 1981.
Decided June 17, 1981.
http://scholar.google.co.uk/scholar_case?case=16807219216043765696&q=OCCUPATIONAL+HEALTH+%26+SAFETY+hazards+not+identified&hl=en&as_sdt=2,5

4. "Environmental disasters as risk regulation catalysts? The role of Bhopal, Chernobyl, Exxon Valdez, Love Canal, and Three Mile Island in shaping U.S. environmental law"
Matthew E. Kahn
Journal of Risk and Uncertainty
August 2007, Volume 35, Issue 1, pp 17-43

5. Disaster Votes
http://superhome.edublogs.org/2010/06/15/disaster-votes/

6 – 9. Environmental disasters reduce likelihood of pro-green votes in Congress
By Phil Hampton, August 17, 2007
http://newsroom.ucla.edu/portal/ucla/Environmental-Disasters-Reduce-8157.aspx

10 – 17. "Nukes in town: Be prepared for all hell to break loose"
Maha Mirza
http://www.skyscrapercity.com/showthread.php?p=91445017

Chapter 12 – Some New Court Decisions – Drowning at Resort

Here's an interesting case, that as cited "Landmark Decision Narrows Application of Occupational Health and Safety Act"

Specifically:

On December 24, 2007, a guest at Blue Mountain Resorts died while swimming in an unattended pool at the resort. When Blue Mountain did not report the incident to the Ministry of Labour, an Inspector concluded that this was a breach of the Occupational Health and Safety Act ("OHSA"), which requires the reporting of any death or critical injury which occurs in a "workplace". Both the Ontario Labour Relations Board (the "Board") and the Divisional Court concluded that the failure to report the incident to a Ministry of Labour Inspector was a breach of the Act because the unattended pool constituted a "workplace", even though there were no workers present at the time.[1]

At issue on appeal was whether a swimming pool at a resort, and by extension, other areas only intermittently frequented by workers, would fit the definition of "workplace" under the OHSA and require reporting of any death or critical injury to the Ministry of Labour.[2]

In setting aside the decisions of the Divisional Court and the Board, the Court of Appeal stated that giving such a broad interpretation to "workplace" under the OHSA would make virtually every place in the province of Ontario a "workplace" because a worker may, at some point in time, be at that place.[3]

The Court of Appeal noted, by way of example, that this interpretation of "workplace" would lead to absurd results, requiring notice to the Ministry of Labour where:
∘A child is injured at home, because the parents have hired a nanny
∘A car accident occurs on a public highway, because the police or other works may arrive after the accident, or may have previously passed by the area
∘A guest dies of a heart attack or is murdered in their hotel room, because hotel employees periodically enter guest rooms[4]

In other words, the Court of Appeal concluded, this interpretation would lead to the absurd conclusion that every death or critical injury to anyone, anywhere in the Province, whatever the cause, would have to be reported. To avoid this absurdity, the Court of Appeal concluded that a proper interpretation of the OHSA is that the reporting obligations only trigger where:
1.A worker or non-worker is killed or critically injured;
2.The death or critical injury occurs at a place where a worker is carrying out his or her employment duties at the time of the incident, or whether the worker might reasonably be expected to be carrying out these duties in the ordinary course of his or her work; and
3.There is a reasonable nexus between the hazard giving rise to the death or critical injury and a realistic risk to worker safety at the workplace.[5]

In the case of Blue Mountain, the Court of Appeal concluded that there was no evidence that the swimming pool death had been caused by any hazard that could affect the safety of a worker.[6]

The actual case is also reported in Appendix 5 and 6, below.

Footnotes

1 – 6. "Landmark Decision Narrows Application of Occupational Health and Safety Act" Mathews, Dinsdale & Clark LLP
http://www.mathewsdinsdale.com/landmark-decision-narrows-application-of-occupational-health-and-safety-act/

Appendix 5

Court Ruling: Every "Person" Counts When Reporting Injuries
Jun 29, 2011
By Jeremy Warning and Cheryl A. Edwards
http://www.healthandsafetyontario.ca/Resources/Articles/WSPS/Court-Ruling--
Every-Person-Counts-When-Reporting.aspx

A skier suffers a broken arm while skiing. A student is knocked unconscious during a physical education class. A patient dies in hospital. Aside from being unfortunate events, incidents such as these are generally not seen as attracting an obligation to report the matter to health and safety authorities. This is no longer the case as a result of a recent OHS decision.

On May 18, 2011, the Ontario Divisional Court upheld an Ontario Labour Relations Board (OLRB) decision that determined that all fatal and critical injuries occurring at a workplace should be reported to the Ministry of Labour. The decision has the potential to significantly impact many Ontario employers and constructors, who are obligated to both report and preserve the scene of the injury as set out in the Occupational Health and Safety Act. The circumstances leading to the decision, its potential ramifications, and practical steps organizations may take to manage their obligations in such cases, are discussed below.

The incident and the order

Blue Mountain Resort Limited operates an inn, ski runs and other recreational facilities on a property of approximately 750 acres. The business employs 1,750 people in peak season. In December 2007, a patron drowned in an unsupervised indoor swimming pool. At the time, no Blue Mountain workers were in the pool area. Blue Mountain did not report the drowning to the Ministry of Labour because it did not involve a worker.

In March 2008, a Ministry of Labour inspector conducting a field visit learned of the drowning and issued an order under subsection 51(1) of the act. The subsection requires that

Where a person is killed or critically injured from any cause at a workplace, the constructor, if any, and the employer shall notify an inspector, and the committee, health and safety representative and trade union, if any, immediately of the occurrence by telephone or other direct means and the employer shall, within forty-eight hours after the occurrence, send to a Director a written report of the circumstances of the occurrence containing such information and particulars as the regulations prescribe.

The order indicated that Blue Mountain had failed to notify an inspector of the "fatal injury to a person" and directed Blue Mountain to comply forthwith, based on the literal wording of this requirement.

The appeal: was a "worker" or "workplace" involved?

Blue Mountain appealed the order to the OLRB, alleging it was incorrect because the drowning incident did not involve a "worker" and/or did not occur in a "workplace." Blue Mountain argued that an interpretation of subsection 51(1) that would require the reporting of injuries sustained by non-workers that occur at a location where no worker is present at the time of the injury is absurd. Blue Mountain asserted that the purpose of the act is to ensure the safety of workers, rather than persons or non-workers, and that the absence of workers from the location of the incident means the location is not a workplace as defined by the act. In taking this position, Blue Mountain argued that the word "person" in subsection 51(1) should be interpreted to mean "worker."

The OLRB upheld the order. While the OLRB agreed that the purpose of the act is to protect workers, it did not agree that "person" means "worker" in subsection 51(1). In reaching this decision, the OLRB considered that the term "person" is not defined in the act, whereas "worker" has a specific defined meaning: "a person who performs work or supplies services for monetary compensation [...]." The OLRB held that a "worker" was a category of "person" and the terms were, therefore, not synonymous. Further the term "person" is broader than the definition of "worker" as it "is generally understood to refer to the broadest range of people."1 The numerous provisions in the act where the term "person" is used establishes that "person" cannot be equated with "worker." In the OLRB's view, had the Legislature intended that employers report only accidents involving workers it would not have used the word "person" in subsection 51(1) of the act.

The OLRB also rejected the argument that, because no Blue Mountain workers were at the pool at the time of the incident, the indoor pool was not a "workplace."2 The OLRB found that Blue Mountain was a fixed workplace; it is a fixed location to which employees regularly report. It had a defined area that consisted of the ski hill, buildings, parking lots and other areas, and that workers employed by Blue Mountain would perform work functions in all or parts of the defined area on a daily basis. The entire 750 acres of the Blue Mountain resort was found to be a "workplace" for the purposes of subsection 51(1). The absence of a worker from a particular location within the defined area did not mean the particular location ceased to be a "workplace." Essentially, the OLRB held that, in a fixed work location like Blue Mountain, areas do not transition in and out of being a "workplace" based on the comings and goings of workers.

The OLRB also declined to interpret subsection 51(1) as only applying to injuries involving workers on policy grounds. It accepted the Ministry of Labour's position that notification of all critical and fatal injuries to all persons is intended because workplace hazards that injure non-workers may also endanger workers.3

Judicial review upholds reporting obligation

Blue Mountain sought judicial review of the OLRB's decision.4 The issues before the Divisional Court were largely the same as were before the OLRB: whether the word "person" in subsection 51(1) should be interpreted to mean "worker" and whether the "workplace" is defined by the physical presence of a worker.

In arriving at its decision, the Court concluded that the OLRB's logic was transparent, intelligible and justified in light of the total context of the legislation's purposes and the language used to implement those purposes. [...] Conditions and hazards that result in the death or critical injury of a non-worker have the potential to cause similar harm to workers. The reporting obligation serves to enhance the protection of workers by bringing hazards to the attention of the ministry whereas an absence of a reporting obligation would lead to a diminished oversight and potentially less worker safety.5

The Court agreed with the OLRB that the physical presence of a worker was not necessary to make a location a "workplace" for the purpose of subsection 51(1). The Court noted that the obligation to report a critical injury or fatality under subsection 51(1) is not entirely based on the timing of the incident but on the "causative nexus between prevailing conditions and the resulting harm."6 The Court agreed that the ministry should be notified of these incidents because the cause may also place workers at risk.

That said, the Court took issue with the OLRB's finding that the entire 750 acre property was a "workplace." The Court held that this finding was unnecessary to resolve the appeal and that each case should be determined on its own merits. Yet, this divergence of opinion did not affect the outcome of the judicial review. The Court found that, notwithstanding the absence of a worker from the swimming pool area at the time of the accident, the area was a "workplace." Consequently, the decision of the OLRB was not unreasonable and the application for judicial review was dismissed.

Blue Mountain Resort Limited is seeking leave to appeal the Divisional Court decision to the Ontario Court of Appeal. Watch for updates in future issues of HSO Network News.

Managing the implications for reporting and preserving the scene

a) Incident reporting. All businesses that provide services to the public at large or other non-workers (such as volunteers) may face the requirement to report fatal and critical consequences involving these persons. We note that subsection 51(1) does not even refer to a fatal or critical injury arising from an incident; rather, the reporting obligation arises if any person is injured from any cause the reporting obligation arises. Subsection 51(1) refers to prompt notification of a ministry inspector, as well as the joint health and safety committee representative and trade union, and then as a second requirement, a written report within 48 hours after the occurrence.

The potential impact on those operating in the retail, hospitality, public transit, education, and other service industries cannot be overstated. Municipal and provincial government bodies operating and maintaining facilities, parks, roads and infrastructure all stand to be significantly impacted. Hospitals, nursing and retirement homes, and provincial jails will now, apparently, have to report every fatality or critical injury occurring within their premises that involves a person such as a patient or inmate. One could reasonably expect that this decision will require almost constant reporting from some employers.

b) Preserving the scene of an incident. Subsection 51(2) requires that the scene of an injury not be disturbed, without the permission of an inspector, except to save life or relieve human suffering, maintain an essential public utility service or a public transportation system, or prevent unnecessary damage to equipment or other property. Blue Mountain had raised this concern before both the OLRB and Divisional Court, noting that it would be required to hold the scene of all incidents involving a critical injury or fatality until released by the ministry. Blue Mountain argued that the requirement to cordon off an incident scene could have a serious impact on their operations. However, the OLRB and the Court did not address this issue as it was not raised on the circumstances of the appeal – which was against an order to report the incident. Without any guidance on this obligation for incidents involving non-workers, employers and constructors must assume that the obligation applies in full, meaning that the scene of an injury will need to be held until released by a ministry inspector.

c) Suggested strategy. In light of the potentially onerous obligations placed on employers and constructors, and the potential consequences of failing to comply with them, short of an amendment to the act or its regulations or a clear policy directive on this matter from the ministry, prompt consideration must be given to managing this issue. All employers and constructors should have in place incident reporting policies, strategies and procedures. In light of the Blue Mountain decision, policies and procedures should be reviewed, and every employer and constructor should be prepared as follows:

1. Clearly state in incident reporting requirements circumstances in which notice and a written report must be given to the ministry, and be amended to reflect reporting where a "person" is killed or critically injured from any cause at a workplace. They should also state circumstances under which the scene should be preserved.

2. Ensure front-line supervisory personnel in workplaces know whom to notify in the event of a fatal or critical injury, and human resources and health and safety personnel have contact information for the ministry available in case notice and a report must be provided. Public and private sector organizations that stand to be significantly affected by the amendments should speak with a regular ministry contact to provide advance notice that increased notifications will be occurring as a result of the Blue Mountain decision.

3. For employers in a sector that will be significantly affected by ongoing incidents potentially giving rise to reporting, keep in mind that the Blue Mountain decision left the door open to a possible argument that a particular event or incident of fatal or critical injury has not occurred at a "workplace." Incident reporting requirements should instruct human resources or OHS personnel to make immediate contact with a local inspector to inquire as to whether the ministry will require notice, a written report, and the preservation of the scene in circumstances where there may not clearly be a notice and reporting obligation. Inquiries of this nature could potentially be made in circumstances involving an incident that
•does not involve an employee or contractor of the organization
•does not arise out of the organization's work or work-related activity
•did not involve the organization's equipment or vehicles
•did not occur in a vehicle, building or area where an employee or contractor of the organization works
•could not readily have happened to an employee or contractor of the organization.

In some instances in the past, the ministry has ruled, upon receiving a verbal notice, that they do not wish a formal notification or report, or the scene to be preserved, where they determine, from the verbal notice, that the matter does not involve a workplace or work-related issue. Such matters should, in the writers' view, be left to the discretion of the ministry. If the ministry does not wish notice, a report or the scene to be preserved, record and retain the name of the ministry official who was contacted.

4.Keep standard letters and reporting forms available, to ensure that minimum statutory notification and written reporting requirements to the ministry, health and safety committee and trade union are met.

While these suggested strategies do not entirely eliminate the possibility that certain organizations will be inundating the ministry with telephone notifications and inquiries, they may help to create an organized, managed approach to the consequences occasioned by this interpretation of subsection 51(1).

Notes

1.1. Blue Mountain Resorts Limited v. Ontario (Labour), 2009 CanLII 13609 at para. 69 (O.L.R.B.).

2. Defined in subsection 1(1) of the act to mean "any land, premises, location or thing at, upon, in or near which a worker works."

3. "I accept the Ministry's submission that, where workers are vulnerable to the same hazards and risks as non-workers who attend at a workplace, it is not an absurd result for an employer to be required to report when a nonworker suffers a critical injury at a workplace. If workers go in or near places where an incident has occurred resulting in a non-worker suffering a critical injury, the workers are equally at risk. The reporting of the nonworker injury serves to enable the Ministry to conduct an investigation and make orders or recommendations designed to enhance the protection of workers". Blue Mountain Resorts Limited v. Ontario (Labour), supra at note 1, at para. 61.

4. There is no ability to appeal a decision of the OLRB. However, an application may be filed with the Divisional Court to have the decision reviewed by the court. A judicial review is different from an appeal as the court will generally focus on whether the OLRB had the authority to make the decision it did and whether it properly exercised that authority. The court will not consider whether it would have made the same decision but will look at whether the decision is reasonable in all of the circumstances.

5. Blue Mountain Resorts Limited v. Ontario (The Ministry of Labour and The Ontario Labour Relations Board, 2011 ONSC 3057 at para. 17 (Ont. S.C.J. (Div. Ct.)).

6. Ibid. at para. 26

Blue Mountain Resorts Limited v. Ontario (The Ministry of Labour and The Ontario Labour Relations Board), 2011 ONSC 3057 (CanLII)

ONTARIO- SUPERIOR COURT OF JUSTICE

DIVISIONAL COURT

J. WILSON, SWINTON AND LOW JJ.

Date: 2011-05-18
Docket: 373/09
http://www.canlii.org/en/on/onscdc/doc/2011/2011onsc3057/2011onsc3057.html

Low J.

[1]   The applicant operates a resort comprising ski runs, an inn and other recreational facilities. The property covers some 750 acres. The business employs about 1,750 workers in peak season. It seeks judicial review of a decision of the Ontario Labour Relations Board ("the Board") dated March 23, 2009 which upheld, on appeal, an order of the respondent Richard Den Bok in his capacity as an inspector under the Occupational Health and Safety Act, 1990, R.S.O. c. O.1, as amended ("the Act").

[2]   The order related to an occurrence at the applicant's premises in which a guest drowned on December 24, 2007, in the unsupervised swimming pool at the resort. The order was made pursuant to s. 51(1) of the Act and arose out of a field visit to the applicant's premises on March 27, 2008.

[3]   Subsection 51(1) of the Act provides:

51. (1) Where a person is killed or critically injured from any cause at a workplace, the constructor, if any, and the employer shall notify an inspector, and the committee, health and safety representative and trade union, if any, immediately of the occurrence by telephone or other direct means and the employer shall, within forty-eight hours after the occurrence, send to a Director a written report of the circumstances of the occurrence containing such information and particulars as the regulations prescribe.

[4]   The inspector concluded that a "person" included a guest, and that a "workplace" included an unsupervised swimming pool. The inspector's order was as follows (at para. 3):

Where a person is killed or critically injured from any cause at a workplace, the constructor, if any, and the employer shall notify an inspector, and the committee, health and safety representative and trade union, if any, immediately of the occurrence by telephone, telegram or other direct means and the employer shall, within forty-eight hours after the occurrence, send to a director a written report of the circumstances of the occurrence containing such information and particulars as the regulations prescribe. THE EMPLOYER FAILED TO NOTIFY AN INSPECTOR OF THE FATAL INJURY TO A PERSON WHICH OCCURRED AT THE BLUE MOUNTAIN INN ON DECEMBER 24, 2007. COMPLY FORTHWITH.

[5]   The applicant believed initially that the guest had suffered a heart attack but it subsequently learned that the guest had drowned. The applicant did not notify an inspector of the occurrence pursuant to s. 51(1) of the Act and did not send to the Director a written report of the circumstances of the occurrence. It was of the view that because the person who drowned was not a worker, the provisions of s. 51(1) of the Act did not apply.

[6]   The Board upheld the inspector's order.

[7]   The two issues before the Board in deciding the applicant's appeal were whether the word "person" in s. 51(1) means "worker" and whether the unsupervised swimming pool in which the guest drowned was a "workplace" within the meaning of the Act.

[8]   "Person" is not defined in the Act.

[9]   "Workplace" is defined in s. 1 as follows:

"workplace" means any land, premises, location or thing at, upon, in or near which a worker works. ("lieu de travail")

[10]   The Board considered the legislative context, the purposes of the Act as set out in R. v. Timminco Ltd., 2001 CanLII 3494 (ON CA), [2001] O.J. No. 1443; 54 O.R. (3d) 21 (C.A.) and Ontario (Ministry of Labour) v. Hamilton (City),2002 CanLII 16893 (ON CA), [2002] O.J. No. 283; 58 O.R. (3d) 37 (C.A.) and the uses of the words "person" and "worker" in different parts of the Act. The Board concluded that the word "person" in s. 51(1) is to be construed in its ordinary meaning and not as synonymous with the word "worker", which is defined in s. 1 of the legislation as

a person who performs work or supplies services for monetary compensation but does not include an inmate of a correctional institution or like institution or facility who participates inside the institution or facility in a work project or rehabilitation program.

[11]   With respect to whether the guest drowned in a "workplace", the Board found the following:

75. Blue Mountain is a fixed workplace. There is a fixed location to which employees regularly report. There is a defined area that encompasses a ski hill, buildings, parking lots, a swimming pool etc. from which Blue Mountain operates its resort. Employees of Blue Mountain move about performing work functions within all or a part of this area on a daily basis. The area of the resort where the Blue Mountain employees perform their work functions is a "workplace" for the purposes of section 51(1) of the Act. The fact that an employee is not physically present within a section of that "workplace" does not mean that that particular section is not part of the "workplace" during the period when no employees are present.

76. I heard no evidence as to the work done by employees of Blue Mountain within the enclosed area of the indoor swimming pool where the guest drowned. I heard no evidence as to how regularly employees go into this area, what they do in the area or how many employees enter this area. However, Blue Mountain did not contest the Ministry's assertion that Blue Mountain employees enter the pool area and did not suggest that persons who were not Blue Mountain employees looked after the pool. Based on general and common knowledge I infer that at least one and perhaps more Blue Mountain employees must enter the enclosed area of the indoor swimming pool in order to clean the pool and check the water at least once, and likely more times, each day. The swimming pool thus comprises a part of at least one Blue Mountain employee's workplace. It does not cease to be a "workplace" because the employee in question moves from that area of his or her workplace to another area of the same workplace.

77. Blue Mountain did not argue that the guest who drowned in the swimming pool had not suffered a critical injury. Although Blue Mountain initially believed the guest had died of natural causes, it subsequently learned that the guest had drowned.

78. For the reasons set out above, I find that the drowning of a guest in the Blue Mountain swimming pool on December 24, 2007 triggered the reporting obligation under subsection 51(1) of the Act, as it involved a "person" who was killed from any cause at a "workplace" ....

[12]   The standard of review on this application is one of reasonableness. The Board is an expert tribunal exercising its powers of decision in the administration of a statute within its area of responsibility (and see also Lennox Drum Ltd. v. Ah-Home, 2010 ONSC 4424 (CanLII), 2010 ONSC 4424 (Div. Ct.)).

[13]   As to the Board's construction of the word "person", the applicant does not challenge the Board's determination that the word is to be given its

plain, ordinary and inclusive meaning. The intervenor, Conservation Ontario, argued that the word "person" should be construed as meaning "worker".

[14]   The applicant and the intervenor raise concerns about the practical application of the reporting requirement flowing from the interpretation of the meaning of "workplace" to include all 750 acres of the entire resort.

[15]   The obligation created by s. 51(1) upon employers to report when a person is killed or critically injured is driven by result rather than by causation. Hence on a plain reading of the subsection, any event resulting in death or critical injury, even if occurring in circumstances having no potential nexus with worker safety, is reportable so long as they occur in a workplace. For purposes of triggering the reporting obligation and ensuring a sufficient reach to deal with incidents having a possibility of genesis in working conditions, the subsection as interpreted by the Board has a potential to reach beyond the ambit of the purposes of the statute.

[16]   The intention to cast a very wide net to ensure that all circumstances resulting in death or critical injury at a workplace are brought to the Ministry's attention is apparent elsewhere in the Act. For example, s. 8(14) provides:

(14) Where a person is killed or critically injured at a workplace from any cause, the health and safety representative may, subject to subsection 51(2), inspect the place where the accident occurred and any machine, device or thing, and shall report his or her findings in writing to a Director. [Emphasis added.]

[17]   The applicant did not challenge in argument the Board's construction of the word "person" as unreasonable. We are of the view that the Board's logic in arriving at that conclusion was transparent, intelligible and justified in light of the total context of the legislation's purposes and the language used to implement those purposes. Nor does it lead to a result that is absurd. Conditions and hazards that result in the death or critical injury of a non-worker have the potential to cause similar harm to workers. The reporting obligation serves to enhance the protection of workers by bringing hazards to the attention of the Ministry whereas an absence of a reporting obligation would lead to a diminished oversight and potentially less worker safety.

[18]   The focus of this application for judicial review is the meaning of "workplace". The manner in which the word "workplace" is to be construed in s. 1 and s. 51(1) raises the same question of the extent of the Act's reach.

[19]   The applicant's position is that the construction of the word "workplace" adopted by the Board leads to an absurd result. The Board held, at paragraph 75, that Blue Mountain is a fixed workplace. Blue Mountain is both a place where some 1,750 individuals work at its peak season and a place of

recreation for many thousands of holiday makers, including skiers in winter and mountain bikers at other times of the year.

[20] The applicant is concerned with the potential for serious disruption to its operations if "person" is construed in its ordinary meaning and "workplace" is defined as the whole of the resort. "Critical injuries" are defined broadly in the regulations to include the fracture of an arm or leg (R.R.O. 1990, Reg. 834, s.1). Because the very nature of skiing is such that injuries, some of them critical as defined in the Act, are an expected and not-infrequent by-product of the activity, a definition of workplace as comprising all of Blue Mountain would, it is argued, result in serious disruption of the resort's operations by reason of the language of s. 51(2) which provides:

(2) Where a person is killed or is critically injured at a workplace, no person shall, except for the purpose of,

(a) saving life or relieving human suffering;

(b) maintaining an essential public utility service or a public transportation system; or

(c) preventing unnecessary damage to equipment or other property,

interfere with, disturb, destroy, alter or carry away any wreckage, article or thing at the scene of or connected with the occurrence until permission so to do has been given by an inspector. [Emphasis added.]

[21] The applicant argues that s. 51(2) requires preservation of the scene of the occurrence and that mischief will ensue because doing so may cause perils to other users of the premises while awaiting permission from the Ministry and because there will be significant disruption to the operation of the recreational facility.

[22] The applicant argues as well, based on the Board's statement at paragraph 75 of the decision, that subject to the statutory exceptions in the Act and premises covered by other legislation, virtually all places are "workplaces" with the result that the Ministry of Labour will have expanded its reach to realms of activity that are completely unrelated to worker health and safety.

[23] Accordingly, it is argued that such a result does not fall within a range of possible, acceptable outcomes which are defensible in respect of the facts and law as described in Dunsmuir v. New Brunswick, 2008 SCC 9 (CanLII), [2008] 1 S.C.R. 190 at para 47.

[24] More specifically, the applicant argues that the Board ought to have

given recognition to the fact that the applicant's facilities are dual use premises –
they are both recreational premises and a workplace and the use may change
depending on the circumstances. A guest may experience a critical injury or be
killed while engaged in a recreational activity on the premises in circumstances
which do not pose a risk to a worker.

[25]   The applicant's position as to the proper construction of the term
"workplace" is one which requires the physical presence of a worker at a place
where a worker works at the time at which an occurrence with a guest or other
person takes place. More specifically, in the instant case, it is the applicant's
position that the swimming pool would have been a workplace had an employee
of the applicant been on site going about his work at the time of the guest
drowning, but no employee being present and working at the time, the swimming
pool was not a workplace when the occurrence took place. Therefore, the
applicant argues, there was no reporting obligation in the facts of this case.

[26]   There are significant logical flaws in the applicant's argument. The
focus is entirely temporal and does not take into account the causative nexus
between prevailing conditions and the resulting harm. For example, had the
swimmer been critically injured by a structural fault in the pool area, it could
hardly be argued that the circumstances ought not to attract the attention of the
Ministry and thus the reporting obligation. Workers and guests are vulnerable to
the same hazards. The purposes and intents of the legislation would be
undermined if a physical hazard with potential to harm workers and non-workers
alike was not subject to reporting and oversight.

[27]   We are of the view that the language of the definition of "workplace"
does not reasonably admit the construction proposed by the applicant. In our
view, had the Legislature intended the construction advanced by the applicant,
the definition of workplace would not be "any land, premises, location or thing at,
upon, in or near which a worker works" but rather "any land...at, upon, in or
near which a worker is working". [Emphasis added.]

[28]   In our view, the applicant's suggested construction is neither
consonant with the language of the definition nor with the purposes of the
legislation.

[29]   That said, we are not persuaded that the Board reasonably concluded
that the whole of the Blue Mountain Resort is a workplace. Such a finding
conflates, in our view, the proprietary interests of the applicant in the 750 acres
of property with the statutory definition of "workplace" and it goes significantly
farther than was necessary for purposes of disposing of the appeal. Each case
must be determined on its own facts.

[30]   In this case, the guest drowned in the resort swimming pool. It is

common ground that the swimming pool is a place where one or more workers work. For these reasons, the absence of a worker at the swimming pool premises at the time of the occurrence does not diminish the fact that it is a workplace, and we are not persuaded that the conclusion reached by the Board was unreasonable.

[31]   Argument was directed to the spectre of disruption of the applicant's operations and of services provided to the public by members of the intervenor if this court were to uphold the Board's holding that "person" means person and "workplace" does not import physical presence of a worker at the time of an occurrence of death or critical injury. Such disruption is said to flow from an obligation under s. 51(2) to preserve the scene of the occurrence. It is suggested that there will be great disruption because the properties operated by the applicant and the intervenor are recreational in nature and attract vast numbers of users who are not workers and who suffer critical injuries in their recreational use of the properties. It is argued that a reporting obligation of such injuries does not advance the purposes of the Act and overexpands the reach of the Ministry of Labour.

[32]   There was no issue before the Board as to whether there had been a failure to comply with s. 51(2) and, in our view, the Board correctly declined to deal with this issue.

[33]   We are of the view that the Board's decision with respect to the obligation to report the swimming pool death was not unreasonable and accordingly dismiss the application.

[34]   The parties are agreed that as this application raises a novel issue, there should be no costs.

Released: May 18, 2011

Chapter 13 – Another Decision – Walmart & Patrick Desjardins

Some of these cases are of interest.

As reported:

Wal-Mart fined $120K in teen's death
 Patrick Desjardins, 17, was electrocuted while buffing floor at Grand Falls store
CBC NewsPosted: Mar 20, 2012
http://www.cbc.ca/news/canada/new-brunswick/wal-mart-fined-120k-in-teen-s-death-
1.1131225

Wal-Mart Canada has been fined $120,000 in connection with the death of a teenaged employee last year in Grand Falls, N.B.

Patrick Desjardins, 17, was electrocuted while using a floor buffing and polishing machine on the wet floor of a garage at the Wal-Mart outlet in the northwestern New Brunswick community on Jan. 5, 2011.

Wal-Mart pleaded guilty Tuesday in Grand Falls provincial court to three charges under the Occupational Health and Safety Act, while supervisor Denis Morin pleaded guilty to two charges under the act.

Crown prosecutor Karen Lee Lamrock said Desjardins' death was neither deliberate nor intentional on the part of Wal-Mart or Morin. It was an accident, resulting from imprudence, not malice or corner-cutting, she said.

"We did not find they have put profit ahead of safety concerns in this case," Lamrock said.

Wal-Mart has taken several remedial steps, the court heard.

Record-setting fine

Patrick Desjardins was electrocuted while buffing the garage floor at the Wal-Mart in Grand Falls, N.B., with an old floor polisher purchased at a yard sale. (CBC)

Still, the Crown asked the court to consider imposing a fine of $100,000 for Wal-Mart, plus a $20,000 victim fine surcharge.

The highest fine ever imposed in New Brunswick for a violation under the act was $30,000, the court heard. But the legislation was changed in 2008, increasing the maximum fine per count to $250,000.

Wal-Mart agreed to the recommended $120,000 fine as part of a joint submission.

Judge Paul Duffie fined the company that amount, saying it was a tragic case, but said he was impressed Wal-Mart had admitted guilt and worked to find a resolution.

Morin, who makes about $36,000 a year, was fined $880, plus a $176 victim fine surcharge, as recommended in the joint submission.

Wal-Mart Canada may be the largest corporation charged by WorkSafeNB, Mike McGovern, a lawyer with the Crown corporation, has said.

Wal-Mart was originally facing a total of eight charges under the act, but those charges were withdrawn and replaced with the three new charges that the company:

■Failed to ensure that the floor polisher was inspected before use and repaired or replaced if necessary, and was maintained in proper working condition, and failed to ensure employees complied with the requirements of tool use.
■Failed to ensure that electrical equipment, including extension cords, were suitable and that they were maintained and modified in accordance to the manufacturer's specifications and appropriately insulated or grounded before each use.
■Failed to take all reasonable precautions to ensure the health and safety of employees by permitting the use of the floor polisher with a faulty extension cord in the tire and lube express area of the store.

The original three charges against Morin were also withdrawn and replaced with two new charges that he:

■Failed to provide a healthy and safe workplace for employees.
■Failed to inform employees of the dangers of using the floor polisher in the garage.

WorkSafeNB laid the original charges following a lengthy investigation.

Floor polisher was purchased at yard sale

Desjardins, a Grade 12 student at John Caldwell School, had been working at Wal-Mart part-time to save money to pay for college. He wanted to become a forest ranger.

His duties included oil changes, tire installations and cleaning the bay floors at the end of the night once the shop was closed, the court heard.

Some of the technicians would use an Electrolux floor polisher, while others would use buckets and mops.

On Jan. 5, 2011, Patrick had been using the floor polisher when he was discovered in the store's garage by another employee at about 8:30 p.m. AT. First aid was administered and the teen was rushed to Grand Falls General Hospital where he was pronounced dead on arrival.

The floor polisher had been purchased by one of the other technicians at a yard sale and brought to the garage for use, the court heard.

Wal-Mart had not authorized its use, so the technicians were not trained to use it and it was not inspected monthly, along with other equipment, the court heard.

But the technician who bought it had been reimbursed for the purchase from the store's petty cash fund and the technicians' supervisor knew it was being used.

Another technician had spliced an extension cord together and spliced it to the buffer. A rag and some green painter's tape were wrapped around the cord.

Video surveillance showed Desjardins' hand came into contact with the rag and the buffer was not plugged into a grounded outlet at the time. His knees buckled, he grabbed the cord and fell onto his back on the wet floor. The polisher fell on top of him and he suffered electrical shock for about 25 seconds before he stopped moving.

Chapter 14 – Another Decision – Worker Cannot Sue for Workplace Injury & the Tragic Case of the Ryan Brothers

Here's an interesting (and tragic) point.

As cited in:

Worker Cannot Sue for Workplace Injury
"Historic trade-off" affirmed
By Earl Phillips on August 6th, 2013
Posted in Employee Obligations, Litigation, Occupational Health and Safety
McCarthy Tétrault LLP, 2013
http://www.bcemployerlaw.com/2013/08/06/worker-cannot-sue-for-workplace-injury/

Workers' rights to sue over workplace accidents are severely restricted by workers compensation schemes across the country. Statutes like the Workers Compensation Act of BC provide workers with access to an insurance scheme that does not depend on finding fault or the ability of the employer to pay for a workplace injury, illness or death. But in exchange, workers cannot sue the employer or other workers. That has been described as the "historic trade-off" and the Supreme Court of Canada recently re-affirmed the principle.

The case of Marine Services International v. Ryan Estate is mostly about the interplay of federal and provincial laws and a full analysis of that issue case can be found on our Canadian Appeals Monitor blog.

For our purposes, the important facts are these:

•The Ryan brothers were drowned when their fishing vessel capsized.
•Marine Services had designed and built the vessel.
•The Ryan brothers were not employees of Marine Services, but they were workers covered by the Newfoundland and Labrador Workplace Health, Safety and Compensation Act.
•Their widows and dependents received compensation under that Act.
•Their estates also sued Marine Services and one of its employees for negligence in the design and construction of the vessel.

Marine Services and its employee argued they could not be sued because of the "historic trade-off" by which the workers compensation legislation prohibited a lawsuit over a workplace death.

The Supreme Court of Canada agreed:

The WHSCA replaces the tort action for negligence with compensation. As such, it is distinct from tort law. Section 44 of the WHSCA provides for the statutory bar that is at the heart of the "historic trade-off".

A direct employment relationship did not exist between the Ryan brothers and Marine Services at the time of the accident that led to their death. However, the statutory bar in s. 44 of the WHSCA does not only benefit an "employer" in a direct employment relationship with the injured worker. Any employer that contributes to the scheme (and any worker of such an employer) benefits from the statutory bar, as long as the worker was injured in the course of his or her employment and injury "occurred … in the conduct of the operations usual in or incidental to the industry carried on by the employer". [paragraphs 31 and 41; emphasis added.]

The BC Workers Compensation Act has essentially the same provisions in section 10. Also, as in Newfoundland and Labrador, the BC Workers Compensation Board is subrogated to the rights of the worker receiving compensation under the Act. That means the Board can pursue an action in the name of the worker. But it should not mean the Board can pursue an action against another employer or worker covered by the Act.

Every now and then there are challenges to the "historic trade-off", but the Marine Services case is the latest affirmation that the principle should hold when an action over a workplace injury, illness or death is brought against an employer or worker covered by the workers compensation scheme.

This case appears below as Appendix 7!

Appendix 7

Marine Services International Ltd. v. Ryan Estate, 2013 SCC 44 (CanLII)
Date: 2013-08-02
Docket: 34429
http://www.canlii.org/en/ca/scc/doc/2013/2013scc44/2013scc44.html?searchUrlHash=A
AAAAQAsTWFyaW5lIFNlcnZpY2VzIEludGVybmF0aW9uYWwgdi4gUnlhbiBFc3Rhd
GUAAAAAAQ

The Ryan brothers died when their ship, the Ryan's Commander, capsized while
returning from a fishing expedition off the coast of Newfoundland and Labrador. Their
widows and dependants (the "Ryan Estates") applied for and received compensation
under Newfoundland and Labrador's Workplace Health, Safety and Compensation Act
("WHSCA"). In addition, proceeding under the federal Maritime Liability Act ("MLA"),
the Ryan Estates commenced an action against Universal Marine Limited, Marine
Services International Limited and its employee P, alleging negligence in the design and
construction of the Ryan's Commander, as well as against the Attorney General of
Canada, alleging negligence in the inspection of the vessel by Transport Canada. Marine
Services and P applied to the Workplace Health, Safety and Compensation Commission
for a determination of whether the action was prohibited by virtue of the statutory bar of
action contained in s. 44 of the WHSCA. The Commission held that the action was
statute barred by s. 44. On judicial review, the Supreme Court, Trial Division,
overturned the decision of the Commission, holding that the doctrines of
interjurisdictional immunity and federal paramountcy applied and therefore that s. 44
must be read down to allow the action to proceed. The majority of the Court of Appeal
upheld the trial judgment.

Held: The appeal should be allowed. Section 44 of the WHSCA is
constitutionally applicable and operative.

The statutory bar at s. 44 of the WHSCA applies on the facts of this case. It
does not only benefit an "employer" in a direct employment relationship with the injured
worker. Any employer that contributes to the scheme and any worker of such an
employer benefits from the statutory bar, as long as the worker was injured in the course
of his or her employment and the injury occurred in the conduct of the operations usual in
or incidental to the industry carried on by the employer. In the case at bar, the
Commission's finding that the injury that led to the death of the Ryan brothers occurred
in the conduct of the operations usual in or incidental to the industry carried on by Marine
Services is entitled to deference. It is a question of mixed fact and law that the
Commission answered by assessing the evidence and interpreting its home statute;
moreover, the WHSCA contains a privative clause. In light of these factors, the standard
of reasonableness applies.

Section 44 of the WHSCA is constitutionally applicable and operative and,
as such, bars the action initiated by the Ryan Estates against Marine Services and P. The

first step in the resolution of a constitutional issue involving the division of powers is an analysis of the "pith and substance" of the impugned legislation, which consists of an inquiry into the true nature of the law in question for the purpose of identifying the matter to which it essentially relates. Then, at the end of a pith and substance analysis, a court should consider interjurisdictional immunity only if there is prior case law favouring its application to the subject matter at hand, as is the case in this appeal. A two‑pronged test must be met to trigger the application of this doctrine. The first step is to determine whether the impugned legislation trenches on the core of a head of power listed in ss. 91 or 92 of the Constitution Act, 1867. Then, if the impugned legislation trenches on the core of a head of power, the second step is to determine whether the encroachment is sufficiently serious. The impugned legislation must impair rather than just affect the core. When interjurisdictional immunity applies, the impugned law is simply inapplicable to the extra‑jurisdictional matter.

Interjurisdictional immunity does not apply in the case at bar. The first prong of the test is met, but not the second. A provincial statute of general application, such as s. 44 of the WHSCA, cannot have the effect of indirectly regulating an issue of maritime negligence law, which is at the core of the federal power over navigation and shipping. By altering the range of claimants who may make use of the statutory maritime negligence action provided by s. 6(2) of the MLA, s. 44 of the WHSCA trenches on the core of the federal power over navigation and shipping. However, s. 44 of the WHSCA does not impair the exercise of the federal power over navigation and shipping. It may affect the exercise of that federal power, however, this level of intrusion is insufficient to trigger interjurisdictional immunity. The intrusion of s. 44 is not significant or serious when one considers the breadth of the federal power over navigation and shipping, the absence of impact on the uniformity of Canadian maritime law, and the historical application of workers' compensation schemes in the maritime context.

The doctrine of federal paramountcy does not apply in this case either, under a proper interpretation of the MLA. According to this doctrine, when the operational effects of provincial legislation are incompatible with federal legislation, the federal legislation must prevail and the provincial legislation is rendered inoperative to the extent of the incompatibility. Federal paramountcy applies where there is an inconsistency between a valid federal legislative enactment and a valid provincial legislative enactment, but not between a common law rule and a valid provincial law. Inconsistency can arise from two different forms of conflict: the operational conflict, when compliance with one statute means a violation of the other statute, and the frustration of federal purpose. The standard for invalidating provincial legislation on the basis of frustration of federal purpose is high.

Section 6(2) of the MLA provides a cause of action to the dependants of a person who dies by the fault or negligence of others in a maritime law context that is to be adjudicated under Canadian maritime law. However, it makes room for the operation of provincial workers' compensation schemes. The WHSCA and the MLA can operate side by side without conflict. Section 6(2) of the MLA provides that a dependant may bring a claim "under circumstances that would have entitled the person, if not deceased, to recover damages". This language suggests that there are situations where a dependant is not allowed to bring an action pursuant to s. 6(2) of the MLA. Such a situation occurs where a statutory provision, such as s. 44 of the WHSCA, prohibits litigation because compensation has already been awarded under a workers' compensation scheme. The statutory bar in s. 44 of the WHSCA removes compensation for workplace injury from the tort system, of which the MLA is a part. As such, for the purposes of s. 6(2) of the MLA, a deceased worker whose dependants are entitled to compensation under the WHSCA is a person who died under circumstances that would not have entitled the worker to recover damages if he or she had lived. The WHSCA, which establishes a no-fault regime to compensate for workplace-related injury, does not frustrate the purpose of s. 6(2) of the MLA, which was enacted to expand the range of claimants who could start an action in maritime negligence law. The WHSCA simply provides for a different regime for compensation that is distinct and separate from tort.

The judgment of the Court was delivered by

LeBel and Karakatsanis JJ. —

I. Introduction and Overview

[1]   The sea took the lives of two fishermen off the coast of Newfoundland and Labrador. Their estates sought compensation in tort from parties allegedly responsible for their death. This appeal raises the issue of whether the statutory bar of action in s. 44 of the Workplace Health, Safety and Compensation Act, R.S.N.L. 1990, c. W-11 (the "WHSCA") applies and bars a negligence action initiated under s. 6(2) of the Marine Liability Act, S.C. 2001, c. 6 (the "MLA"). The widows and dependants of the deceased fishermen commenced the action after having received compensation under the WHSCA.

[2]   The majority of the Court of Appeal found that the statutory bar in s. 44 of the WHSCA was inapplicable due to interjurisdictional immunity and inoperative by virtue of federal paramountcy.

[3]   We would allow the appeal. Section 44 of the WHSCA applies and it is both constitutionally applicable and operative. The negligence action is therefore dismissed.

II. Background Facts

[4]   Joseph and David Ryan (the "Ryan brothers") tragically died on September 19, 2004 when their ship, the Ryan's Commander, capsized while returning from a fishing expedition off the coast of Newfoundland and Labrador. Their widows and dependants (the "Ryan Estates") applied for and received compensation under the WHSCA.

[5]   Proceeding under the MLA, the Ryan Estates also commenced an action in 2006 against Universal Marine Limited ("Universal Marine"), Marine Services International Limited ("Marine Services") and its employee David Porter, alleging negligence in the design and construction of the Ryan's Commander, which had been commissioned by the Ryan brothers in 2003. The action was also brought against the Attorney General of Canada, alleging negligence in the inspection of the vessel by Transport Canada. If the negligence action were to succeed, the Ryan Estates have indicated that the Workplace Health, Safety and Compensation Commission (the "Commission") would seek repayment of the compensation received by the Ryan Estates under the WHSCA.

[6]   Marine Services and Mr. Porter applied to the Commission under s. 46 of the WHSCA for a determination of whether the Ryan Estates' action is prohibited by virtue of the statutory bar in s. 44 of the WHSCA. The Commission held that the action was statute barred by s. 44. According to the Commission, the WHSCA applied because the Ryan brothers had died in the course of their employment, and Universal Marine, Marine Services, and the Attorney General of Canada were "employers" and David Porter was a "worker" within the meaning of s. 2 of the WHSCA. The Commission concluded that the constitutional doctrines of interjurisdictional immunity and federal paramountcy did not apply.

III. Judicial History

A. Supreme Court of Newfoundland and Labrador — Trial Division (Hall J.), 2009 NLTD 120 (CanLII), 2009 NLTD 120, 289 Nfld. & P.E.I.R. 198

[7]   On judicial review, Hall J. overturned the decision of the Commission. He determined that the WHSCA is, in pith and substance, an insurance scheme. He also held that liability in the marine context falls within the exclusive federal jurisdiction over "Navigation and Shipping" under s. 91(10) of the Constitution Act, 1867. He found that the right to make a claim under the MLA is a core feature of that federal power.

[8]   Hall J. held that interjurisdictional immunity applied. In his opinion, the statutory bar in s. 44 of the WHSCA impaired the right to make a claim under the MLA, which belongs to the core of the federal power over navigation and shipping. He therefore concluded that s. 44 must be read down so as not to bar the action initiated by the Ryan Estates.

[9]   Hall J. also determined that federal paramountcy applied because the Ryan Estates could not comply with both the MLA and the WHSCA. This conflict required that s. 44 of the WHSCA be read down to allow the action of the Ryan Estates to proceed. At the judicial review hearing, the parties agreed that the Attorney General of Canada was not an employer under the WHSCA.

B. Supreme Court of Newfoundland and Labrador — Court of Appeal (Green C.J.N.L. and Welsh and Rowe JJ.A.), 2011 NLCA 42 (CanLII), 2011 NLCA 42, 308 Nfld. & P.E.I.R. 1

[10]   The majority of the Court of Appeal upheld the trial judgment. It noted that Parliament and the legislature chose to enact "two fundamentally different legal regimes dealing with compensation for injury and death, and [that] these two regimes appear to overlap in their application to claims arising out of workplace injuries in a marine environment" (para. 54). It also noted that the MLA adopts a fault-based approach, whereas the WHSCA establishes a no-fault insurance scheme.

[11]   The majority held that the WHSCA is a valid exercise of the provincial power over property and civil rights under s. 92(13) of the Constitution Act, 1867. However, interjurisdictional immunity applied because s. 44 of the WHSCA trenches on maritime negligence law, which sits at the core of the federal power over navigation and shipping: Ordon Estate v. Grail, 1998 CanLII 771 (SCC), [1998] 3 S.C.R. 437. Since s. 44 of the WHSCA purports to bar an action based on maritime negligence law, it impairs the core of that federal power.

[12]   The majority also concluded that federal paramountcy applied. It explained that an operational conflict arose between the MLA and the WHSCA because a maritime claimant who is subject to the WHSCA could bring an action under the MLA. The majority held that the words "circumstances that would have entitled the person, if not deceased, to recover damages" in s. 6(2) of the MLA cannot reasonably be interpreted as allowing provincial workers' compensation legislation to determine the scope of the right to access the federal maritime tort regime. Even if dual compliance was possible, the operation of s. 44 frustrated the purpose of the MLA by denying access to the federal maritime tort regime to the dependants of persons who die in maritime incidents.

[13]   In dissent, Welsh J.A. concluded that federal paramountcy did not apply. She was of the view that no operational conflict arose between s. 6(2) of the MLA and s. 44 of the WHSCA. In her opinion, while the latter takes away the right of the deceased person to sue to recover damages, the former simply says that the dependants "may" start an action "under circumstances" where the deceased would have been entitled to do so. She explained that a liberal interpretation of the MLA allows for dependants of a deceased person to start an action unless, in the circumstances, an action to recover damages is not available for a statutory reason. Such a statutory reason exists in this case, as the entitlement to compensation under the WHSCA precludes the deceased's entitlement to sue. This interpretation permits compliance with both statutes. Furthermore, she was of the view that the fact that s. 44 of the WHSCA restricts the scope of the right granted under s. 6(2) of the MLA is not sufficient to establish the frustration of a federal purpose.

[14]   Welsh J.A. also held that interjurisdictional immunity did not apply because s. 44 of the WHSCA does not trench on the core of the federal power over navigation and shipping. She determined that the WHSCA is a workers' compensation scheme which does not engage issues of negligence. As such, the rationale underlying this Court's determination in Ordon, i.e. that maritime negligence law is a core element of federal jurisdiction over navigation and shipping, does not apply to workers' compensation legislation.

IV. Analysis

A. Issues

[15]   In this appeal, two issues must be addressed. First, does s. 44 of the WHSCA apply on the facts of this case? Second, if s. 44 applies, is it constitutionally applicable and operative? Regarding the second issue, the Chief Justice formulated two constitutional questions:

1. Is s. 44 of the Workplace Health, Safety and Compensation Act, R.S.N.L. 1990, c. W-11, constitutionally inoperative in respect of federal maritime negligence claims made pursuant to s. 6 of the Marine Liability Act, S.C. 2001, c. 6, by reason of the doctrine of federal paramountcy?

2. Is s. 44 of the Workplace Health, Safety and Compensation Act, R.S.N.L. 1990, c. W-11, constitutionally inapplicable to federal maritime negligence claims made pursuant to s. 6 of the Marine Liability Act, S.C. 2001, c. 6, by reason of the doctrine of interjurisdictional immunity?

B. Relevant Legislative Provisions

[16]   Two legislative provisions are relevant to this appeal: s. 44 of the WHSCA and s. 6(2) of the MLA. Section 44 of the WHSCA provides as follows:

44.   (1) The right to compensation provided by this Act is instead of rights and rights of action, statutory or otherwise, to which a worker or his or her dependents are entitled against an employer or a worker because of an injury in respect of which compensation is payable or which arises in the course of the worker's employment.

(2)   A worker, his or her personal representative, his or her dependents or the employer of the worker has no right of action in respect of an injury against an employer or against a worker of that employer unless the injury occurred otherwise than in the conduct of the operations usual in or incidental to the industry carried on by the employer.

(3)   An action does not lie for the recovery of compensation under this Act and claims for compensation shall be determined by the commission.

[17]   Section 6(2) of the MLA provides as follows:

6. . . .

(2)   If a person dies by the fault or neglect of another under circumstances that would have entitled the person, if not deceased, to recover damages, the dependants of the deceased person may maintain an action in a court of competent jurisdiction for their loss resulting from the death against the person from whom the deceased person would have been entitled to recover.

C. Positions of the Parties

   (1)   Application of Section 44 of the WHSCA

[18]   The first issue is the interpretation of the WHSCA and the determination of its scope of application. Only the Ryan Estates address this issue in their factum before this Court. However, the issue was discussed at length at the hearing. The appellants submit that s. 44 of the WHSCA applies and bars the action initiated by the Ryan Estates for the reasons stated by the Commission: the appellants are subject to the WHSCA, the Ryan brothers were injured in the course of their employment, and "the injury occurred ... in the conduct of the operations usual in or incidental to the industry carried on by" Marine Services. The Ryan Estates respond that s. 44 does not apply because the Ryan brothers were not employed by Marine Services at the time of the accident that caused their death. The Attorney General of Canada made no submissions on this issue.

   (2)   Constitutional Applicability and Operability of Section 44 of the WHSCA

      (i)   Interjurisdictional Immunity

[19]   Assuming that s. 44 applies, the parties then address the second issue: the constitutional applicability and operability of s. 44. The appellants submit that the doctrine of interjurisdictional immunity is not engaged. The statutory bar in the WHSCA applies only to employers and workers in one province. It does not impair the uniformity of Canadian maritime law. Canadian law has long recognized the application of provincial workers' compensation legislation in the maritime context. The Court of Appeal erred in its application of this Court's decision in Ordon. The judgment of our Court held that maritime negligence law is at the core of the federal power over navigation and shipping and that it is constitutionally impermissible for a provincial statute of general application to indirectly regulate maritime negligence law issues. But, unlike Ordon, this case concerns the nature of the civil rights as between provincial

employers and workers. Federal jurisdiction over navigation and shipping is not engaged and should not preclude the operation of provincial workers' compensation schemes in maritime industries.

[20]   The Ryan Estates say that the doctrine of interjurisdictional immunity is triggered. Maritime negligence law belongs to the core of the federal competence over navigation and shipping. The WHSCA indirectly regulates maritime negligence law by eliminating recourse to a statutory maritime negligence action. Eliminating access to the right of the action provided by s. 6(2) of the MLA seriously impairs this core and triggers the application of the doctrine of interjurisdictional immunity.

[21]   The Attorney General of Canada also submits that interjurisdictional immunity applies. Maritime negligence law, which is part of the core of federal jurisdiction over navigation and shipping, includes the rules relating to who can be compensated for death and injury resulting from a maritime accident. The statutory bar in s. 44 of the WHSCA sterilizes the right of dependants to sue for wrongful death pursuant to s. 6(2) of the MLA. There is no higher form of impairment.

(ii)   Federal Paramountcy

[22]   The parties also address the other constitutional issue, the application of the doctrine of federal paramountcy. The appellants argue that paramountcy does not apply. The federal and provincial statutes can operate together without conflict because there is no right to make a claim pursuant to s. 6(2) of the MLA where a fatality occurs "under circumstances" that deny to the deceased person the right to recover damages under the general liability regime (for example where, as here, litigation is barred by a provincial workers' compensation scheme). Moreover, the fact that the provincial statute limits the scope of the right under s. 6(2) of the MLA does not frustrate a federal purpose.

[23]   The Ryan Estates submit that paramountcy applies. First, an operational conflict exists if s. 44 of the WHSCA bars an action against any employer that is subject to the scheme. Then, the Ryan Estates say that the provision frustrates the federal purpose of regulating marine liability claims by eliminating recourse to the MLA. The application of that provincial bar would have far-reaching implications for liability claims under the MLA. An "employer" would not be subject to federal marine liability in certain instances because of the protection granted to it under provincial law.

[24]   The Attorney General of Canada agrees with the Ryan Estates. Section 6(2) of the MLA is the gateway to the federal maritime tort regime for dependants of seamen who die at sea. Parliament determined that dependants can maintain any maritime liability action that would have been available to the deceased person. The statutory bar in the provincial statute denies them that cause of action. The two laws are diametrically opposed; the one extinguishes the other. Moreover, the provincial law frustrates the federal purpose of creating a cause of action that allows

dependants to choose their preferred method of obtaining compensation after a wrongful death in the maritime context and maintaining national uniformity in maritime negligence law.

(3) Interveners

[25]   The interveners are the Attorneys General of Ontario, Nova Scotia, British Columbia and Newfoundland and Labrador, the Newfoundland and Labrador Workplace Health, Safety and Compensation Commission, and the Workers' Compensation Board of British Columbia. Collectively, the interveners agree with the appellants that s. 44 of the WHSCA applies and that the provision engages neither federal paramountcy nor interjurisdictional immunity.

D. Nature of Workers' Compensation Schemes

[26]   Professor Peter Hogg concisely describes the general nature and operation of workers' compensation schemes:

Workers' compensation is a public insurance plan that provides compensation for workers injured by accident in the course of their employment. It is financed by premiums paid by employers under compulsion of law, and it is administered by a public agency, usually called a Workers' Compensation Board. The benefits are payable for all work-related accidents (and some occupational diseases are now usually covered as well) regardless of whether or not there was negligence on the part of the employer. In all provinces and territories, the common law action for negligence has been abolished for work-related injuries, leaving the statutory scheme as the exclusive source of compensation.

(P. W. Hogg, Constitutional Law of Canada (5th ed. Supp.), vol. 1, at p. 33-9)

[27]   Provincial workers' compensation schemes generally cover persons employed in the relevant province, even if a workplace accident occurs outside of the province: Workmen's Compensation Board v. Canadian Pacific Railway Co., [1920] A.C. 184 (P.C.) ("Canadian Pacific Railway"). The compensatory elements of these schemes apply to federal undertakings operating within the province, but the occupational health and safety elements do not: Bell Canada v. Quebec (Commission de la santé et de la sécurité du travail), 1988 CanLII 81 (SCC), [1988] 1 S.C.R. 749, at p. 763 and Tessier Ltée v. Quebec (Commission de la santé et de la sécurité du travail), 2012 SCC 23 (CanLII), 2012 SCC 23, [2012] 2 S.C.R. 3, at paras. 5-6.

[28]   Workers' compensation schemes in Canada are rooted in a report by the Honourable Sir William Ralph Meredith, former Chief Justice of Ontario, who was appointed in 1910 to study approaches to workers' compensation and to recommend a scheme for Ontario. In 1914, Ontario adopted his proposal to compensate "injured

workers through an accident fund collected from industry and under the management of the state", and the other provinces followed: Hogg, at p. 33-9, Pasiechnyk v. Saskatchewan (Workers' Compensation Board), 1997 CanLII 316 (SCC), [1997] 2 S.C.R. 890, at para. 24.

[29]   The central element of Sir Meredith's proposal was what has come to be called the "historic trade-off": workers "lost their cause of action against their employers but gained compensation that depends neither on the fault of the employer nor its ability to pay", while employers had to contribute to a common fund "but gained freedom from potentially crippling liability": Pasiechnyk, at para. 25.

[30]   This "historic trade-off" provides timely and guaranteed compensation for workers (or their dependants) and reduces liability for employers. In Pasiechnyk, Sopinka J. described it as a necessary and central feature to a workers' compensation scheme (para. 26). See also Reference re: Workers' Compensation Act, 1983 (Nfld.), ss. 32, 34 1987 CanLII 118 (NL CA), (1987), 44 D.L.R. (4th) 501 (Nfld. C.A.).

[31]   The WHSCA is a workers' compensation scheme in Newfoundland and Labrador providing no-fault compensation to workers and their dependants arising from workplace accidents; it mandates automatic compensation without the need to establish fault on the part of the employer. The WHSCA replaces the tort action for negligence with compensation. As such, it is distinct from tort law. Section 44 of the WHSCA provides for the statutory bar that is at the heart of the "historic trade-off".

[32]   Workers' compensation schemes, which concern employment and insurance law, fall within provincial jurisdiction over property and civil rights as provided by s. 92(13) of the Constitution Act, 1867: see Canadian Pacific Railway; Commission du salaire minimum v. Bell Telephone Co. of Canada, 1966 CanLII 1 (SCC), [1966] S.C.R. 767; Bell Canada; Alltrans Express Ltd. v. British Columbia (Workers' Compensation Board), 1988 CanLII 83 (SCC), [1988] 1 S.C.R. 897; and Husky Oil Operations Ltd. v. Minister of National Revenue, 1995 CanLII 69 (SCC), [1995] 3 S.C.R. 453, at para. 117 per Iacobucci J., dissenting. In Canadian Pacific Railway, the Privy Council said the following about the British Columbia Workmen's Compensation Act, R.S.B.C. 1916, c. 77 (p. 191):

The scheme of the Act is not one for interfering with rights outside the Province. It is in substance a scheme for securing a civil right within the Province.

[33]   Parliament has also adopted two workers' compensation schemes based on the Meredith model: the Government Employees Compensation Act, R.S.C. 1985, c. G-5 (the "GECA"), and the Merchant Seamen Compensation Act, R.S.C. 1985, c. M-6 (the "MSCA"). The first statute was adopted pursuant to Parliament's exclusive jurisdiction over federal employees under s. 91(8) of the Constitution Act, 1867: Attorney General of Canada v. St. Hubert Base Teachers' Association, 1983 CanLII 131 (SCC),

[1983] 1 S.C.R. 498; Société canadienne des postes v. Commission d'appel en matière de lésions professionnelles, 1999 CanLII 13745 (QC CA), [1999] R.J.Q. 957 (C.A.), at pp. 962-63; and Société canadienne des postes v. Commission de la santé et de la sécurité du travail, 1996 CanLII 6426 (QC CA), [1996] R.J.Q. 873 (C.A.), at p. 876. The second statute was an exercise of Parliament's jurisdiction over navigation and shipping. We will briefly review those two statutes to highlight the similarities between them and the WHSCA.

[34]   The GECA applies to individuals working in any capacity for the federal government with the exception of the regular members of the Canadian Forces or the Royal Canadian Mounted Police: ss. 2 ("employee") and 3(1). Section 12 provides that where an accident happens to an employee in the course of his or her employment under circumstances that entitle the employee or his or her dependants to compensation under the GECA, neither the employee nor the dependants "has any claim against Her Majesty, or any officer, servant or agent of Her Majesty". Section 9(1) says that where an accident happens to an employee in the course of his or her employment under circumstances that entitle the employee or the dependants "to an action against a person other than Her Majesty", the employee or the dependants may elect between compensation under the GECA or "may claim against that other person" (s. 45(1) of the WHSCA provides similar election rights to s. 9(1) of the GECA).

[35]   Like the WHSCA, the GECA is a no-fault regime that provides for compensation in case of injury or death caused during employment. A central feature of that no-fault regime is the bar on claims against Her Majesty, which is the employer for employees covered by the GECA.

[36]   The other statute, the MSCA, applies to seamen engaged in home-trade and foreign voyages. The definition of "seaman" excludes fishers, pilots, and apprenticed pilots: s. 2(1). An "employer" under the MSCA "includes every person having any seaman in his service under a contract of hiring or apprenticeship, written or oral, express or implied": s. 2(1). The MSCA does not apply and no compensation is payable under it where a seaman is "entitled to claim compensation under the [GECA] or under any provincial workers' compensation law": s. 5(a).

[37]   In one respect, the MSCA differs from the GECA or provincial workers' compensation regimes such as the WHSCA. Whereas, in the case of the WHSCA, employers must contribute to a collective insurance fund based on assessment (there is no such fund for the GECA as Her Majesty is the only employer), s. 30(1) of the MSCA requires employers to "cover by insurance or other means satisfactory to the [Merchant Seaman Compensation] Board the risks of compensation arising under this Act". Such employers do not contribute to a shared insurance fund, but they must nonetheless obtain insurance.

[38]   In other respects, the MSCA is similar to other workers' compensation schemes: the employer must pay compensation on a no-fault basis (s. 8)

and the right to compensation is in lieu of all rights of action of a seaman or his dependants against the employer (s. 13). Therefore, the historic trade-off of compensation in lieu of a right to sue is, like for the GECA and provincial workers' compensation schemes, at the heart of the MSCA. The MSCA also allows seamen to claim compensation under it or to bring an action against a third party, i.e. a "person other than his co-employees, his employer, the servants or mandataries of his employer": s. 24(1). However, "[n]o seaman entitled to compensation under [the MSCA] or the dependants of the seaman have a right of action against an employer who is subject to [the MSCA]": s. 24(5).

[39]   The above review of the GECA and the MSCA highlights their similarities with the WHSCA and their nature as no-fault insurance schemes for workplace-related injury. Despite some differences, all of these statutes provide compensation in lieu of the right to bring an action; this is the historic trade-off at the heart of the Meredith model of workers' compensation schemes. By establishing no-fault schemes for workplace-related injuries, these statutes are distinct from and do not interact with any tort regimes.

E.   Application of Section 44 of the WHSCA

[40]   Before engaging in a constitutional analysis of whether s. 44 of the WHSCA is applicable and operative, we must first determine if the facts of this case give rise to its application. The Ryan Estates submit that s. 44 does not apply because the Ryan brothers were not employed by Marine Services when the accident that caused their death occurred. We disagree. We are of the view that s. 44 of the WHSCA applies on the facts of this case. As a result, constitutional issues arise and must be resolved.

[41]   A direct employment relationship did not exist between the Ryan brothers and Marine Services at the time of the accident that led to their death. However, the statutory bar in s. 44 of the WHSCA does not only benefit an "employer" in a direct employment relationship with the injured worker. Any employer that contributes to the scheme (and any worker of such an employer) benefits from the statutory bar, as long as the worker was injured in the course of his or her employment and the injury "occurred ... in the conduct of the operations usual in or incidental to the industry carried on by the employer". The Commission assesses, levies, and collects contribution to the injury fund from employers that are subject to the WHSCA, all of whom are obligated to contribute: ss. 97 and 99. Unless excluded by regulation, the WHSCA applies to employers "engaged in, about or in connection with an industry in the province": s. 38(1) ("employer" is also defined in s. 2(j) of the WHSCA).

[42]   The parties do not dispute the Commission's findings that: (a) the Ryan brothers were injured in the course of employment within the meaning of the WHSCA; (b) Marine Services is an "employer" under the WHSCA; and (c) David Porter is a "worker" under the WHSCA.

[43]   The dispute is whether the injury that led to the Ryan brothers' death "occurred otherwise than in the conduct of the operations usual in or incidental to the industry carried on by the employer" as stated in s. 44(2). The answer to this question determines whether s. 44 of the WHSCA applies to this case.

[44]   At the Commission, Marine Services submitted that it was engaged "in operations connected to the fishing industry", "in the business of marine consulting, naval architecture, and vessel design", and that David Porter was, at the relevant time, employed by it to design the vessel (A.R., at p. 17). The Commission agreed with these submissions in its findings of fact (pp. 28-29). On the question of whether the death of the Ryan brothers "occurred ... in the conduct of the operations usual in or incidental to the industry carried on by the employer", the Commission found that it clearly occurred in such a manner (p. 29).

[45]   This appeal is from a judicial review of the Commission's decision. The Commission's finding that the injury that led to the death of the Ryan brothers occurred "in the conduct of the operations usual in or incidental to the industry carried on" by Marine Services is entitled to deference. It is a question of mixed fact and law that the Commission answered by assessing the evidence and interpreting its home statute. Moreover, s. 19 of the WHSCA contains a privative clause. In light of these factors, the standard of reasonableness applies: Dunsmuir v. New Brunswick, 2008 SCC 9 (CanLII), 2008 SCC 9, [2008] 1 S.C.R. 190, at paras. 52-55. On this standard, the Commission's finding should not be disturbed.

[46]   Therefore, s. 44 of the WHSCA applies to this case and, if constitutionally applicable and operative, bars the action initiated by the Ryan Estates against the appellants. We must now turn to the constitutional questions raised by the application of s. 44.

F.   Constitutional Questions

[47]   The constitutional issue is whether a statutory bar of action in a provincial workers' compensation scheme can preclude a person to whom the bar applies from bringing a negligence action that is provided for by a federal maritime negligence statute. The constitutional dispute in this appeal, therefore, concerns the division of powers between the federal and provincial governments under the Constitution Act, 1867.

[48]   The first step in the resolution of a constitutional issue involving the division of powers is an analysis of the "pith and substance" of the impugned legislation: Canadian Western Bank v. Alberta, 2007 SCC 22 (CanLII), 2007 SCC 22, [2007] 2 S.C.R. 3, at para. 25. The analysis of the pith and substance consists of "an inquiry into the true nature of the law in question for the purpose of identifying the 'matter' to which it essentially relates": Canadian Western Bank, at para. 26. Two aspects of the law or of the impugned provision are analyzed: the purpose of the enacting body in adopting it, and

the legal effect of the law or provision: Canadian Western Bank, at para. 27. In this case, the validity of the WHSCA (and of the MLA for that matter) is not contested and a full pith and substance analysis is not required.

[49]   At the end of a pith and substance analysis, a court should generally consider interjurisdictional immunity only if there is "prior case law favouring its application to the subject matter at hand": Canadian Western Bank, at para. 78. The doctrine "is of limited application and should in general be reserved for situations already covered by precedent": Canadian Western Bank, at para. 77. In view of this Court's decision in Ordon, we must consider whether interjurisdictional immunity applies. After conducting that analysis, we will proceed to the determination of whether federal paramountcy applies. For the reasons that follow, we conclude that neither interjurisdictional immunity nor federal paramountcy applies in this case and that s. 44 of the WHSCA is thus constitutionally applicable and operative.

(1)   Interjurisdictional Immunity

[50]   Interjurisdictional immunity exists to protect the "basic, minimum and unassailable content" or the core of the "exclusive classes of subject" created by ss. 91 and 92 of the Constitution Act, 1867: Bell Canada, at p. 839. This Court discussed interjurisdictional immunity in Canadian Western Bank and later in Quebec (Attorney General) v. Canadian Owners and Pilots Association, 2010 SCC 39 (CanLII), 2010 SCC 39, [2010] 2 S.C.R. 536 ("COPA"). The doctrine has a limited application today: Canadian Western Bank, at paras. 33-34. In General Motors of Canada Ltd. v. City National Leasing, 1989 CanLII 133 (SCC), [1989] 1 S.C.R. 641, Dickson C.J. stated that the dominant tide of constitutional interpretation, which favours, where possible, the operation of statutes enacted by both levels of government, militates against interjurisdictional immunity. A broad application of the doctrine is inconsistent with a flexible and pragmatic approach to federalism. As stated earlier, interjurisdictional immunity "is of limited application and should in general be reserved for situations already covered by precedent": Canadian Western Bank, at para. 77.

[51]   There is prior case law favouring the application of interjurisdictional immunity to the subject matter of this appeal. In Ordon, this Court considered negligence claims related to two boating accidents that resulted in death and injury. Since the accidents occurred in navigable waters, the Canada Shipping Act, R.S.C. 1985, c. S-9, applied. However, the plaintiffs relied on Ontario statutes permitting a) negligence claims to be brought by siblings of a deceased or injured victim; b) the recovery of damages for the loss of guidance, care and companionship of a deceased or injured victim; and c) apportionment of damages in cases of contributory negligence, as these options were not available under the Canada Shipping Act.

[52]   This Court concluded that maritime negligence law is part of the core of the federal power over "Navigation and Shipping" under s. 91(10) of the Constitution Act, 1867, and that interjurisdictional immunity will apply if a provincial statute of

general application has the effect of indirectly regulating a maritime negligence law issue. Iacobucci and Major JJ. stated the following, at paras. 84-85:

Maritime negligence law is a core element of Parliament's jurisdiction over maritime law. The determination of the standard, elements, and terms of liability for negligence between vessels or those responsible for vessels has long been an essential aspect of maritime law, and the assignment of exclusive federal jurisdiction over navigation and shipping was undoubtedly intended to preclude provincial jurisdiction over maritime negligence law, among other maritime matters. As discussed below, there are strong reasons to desire uniformity in Canadian maritime negligence law. Moreover, the specialized rules and principles of admiralty law deal with negligence on the waters in a unique manner, focussing on concerns of "good seamanship" and other peculiarly maritime issues. Maritime negligence law may be understood, in the words of Beetz J. in Bell Canada v. Quebec, supra, at p. 762, as part of that which makes maritime law "specifically of federal jurisdiction".

In our opinion, where the application of a provincial statute of general application would have the effect of regulating indirectly an issue of maritime negligence law, this is an intrusion upon the unassailable core of federal maritime law and as such is constitutionally impermissible. . . . In the context of an action arising from a collision between boats or some other accident, maritime negligence law encompasses the following issues, among others: the range of possible claimants, the scope of available damages, and the availability of a regime of apportionment of liability according to fault. A provincial statute of general application dealing with such matters within the scope of the province's legitimate powers cannot apply to a maritime law negligence action, and must be read down to achieve this end.

[53]   Like Ordon, the present appeal involves the reliance by one of the parties on provincial law in relation to a maritime negligence action.

[54]   In COPA, at para. 27, McLachlin C.J. enunciated a two-pronged test that must be met to trigger the application of the doctrine of interjurisdictional immunity:

The first step is to determine whether the provincial law — s. 26 of the Act — trenches on the protected "core" of a federal competence. If it does, the second step is to determine whether the provincial law's effect on the exercise of the protected federal power is sufficiently serious to invoke the doctrine of interjurisdictional immunity. [Emphasis in original.]

[55]   Therefore, we must first consider whether the impugned legislation trenches on the core of a head of power listed in ss. 91 or 92 of the Constitution Act, 1867. Here, the jurisprudence serves as a useful guide to identify the core of a head of power: Canadian Western Bank, at para. 77; COPA, at para. 36.

[56]   Then, if the impugned legislation trenches on the core of a head of power, we must determine whether the encroachment is sufficiently serious. Rather than just "affect" the core, the impugned legislation must "impair" it for interjurisdictional immunity to apply: "the former does not imply any adverse consequence whereas the latter does": Canadian Western Bank, at para. 48. In that case, the majority explained, at para. 48:

It is when the adverse impact of a law adopted by one level of government increases in severity from "affecting" to "impairing" (without necessarily "sterilizing" or "paralyzing") that the "core" competence of the other level of government (or the vital or essential part of an undertaking it duly constitutes) is placed in jeopardy, and not before.

To the same effect, McLachlin C.J. stated in COPA that "impairment" is a higher standard than "affects", as in "an era of cooperative, flexible federalism, application of the doctrine of interjurisdictional immunity requires a significant or serious intrusion on the exercise" of a head of power: para. 45.

[57]   When interjurisdictional immunity applies, the impugned law is not rendered invalid; it is "simply inapplicable to the extra-jurisdictional matter", and it is read down to limit the scope of its application: Hogg, at 15-28 (emphasis in original).

[58]   The Ryan Estates contend (and the majority of the Court of Appeal agreed) that interjurisdictional immunity applies because s. 44 of the WHSCA eliminates the Ryan Estates' access to s. 6(2) of the MLA, a statutory expression of maritime negligence law. They add that this Court decided in Ordon that maritime negligence law is at the core of the federal power over navigation and shipping.

[59]   Maritime negligence law is indeed at the core of the federal power over navigation and shipping: Ordon, at para. 84. A provincial statute of general application cannot have the effect of indirectly regulating an issue of maritime negligence law, such as the range of possible claimants in a maritime negligence action: Ordon, at para. 85. Section 44 of the WHSCA, a provincial statute of general application, precludes the Ryan Estates from making use of the maritime negligence action provided by s. 6(2) of the MLA. By altering the range of claimants who may make use of this statutory maritime negligence action, s. 44 of the WHSCA trenches on the core of the federal power over navigation and shipping. The first prong of the test is therefore met.

[60]   However, we conclude that the second prong of the test is not met as s. 44 of the WHSCA does not impair the exercise of the federal power over navigation and shipping. At para. 45 of COPA, McLachlin C.J. described impairment as suggesting

an impact that not only affects the core federal power, but does so in a way that seriously or significantly trammels the federal power. In an era of cooperative, flexible federalism, application of the doctrine of interjurisdictional immunity requires a significant or serious intrusion on the exercise of the federal power. It need not paralyze it, but it must be serious.

[61]　　　　　Parliament's exclusive legislative jurisdiction over navigation and shipping is broad: Queddy River Driving Boom Co. v. Davidson (1883), 10 S.C.R. 222; and Montreal City v. Montreal Harbour Commissioners, [1926] A.C. 299 (P.C.). It "encompasses those aspects of navigation and shipping that engage national concerns which must be uniformly regulated across the country, regardless of their territorial scope" (Tessier, at para. 22), and includes "maritime law which establishes the framework of legal relationships arising out of navigation and shipping activities" and "the infrastructure of navigation and shipping activities": British Columbia (Attorney General) v. Lafarge Canada Inc., 2007 SCC 23 (CanLII), 2007 SCC 23, [2007] 2 S.C.R. 86, at para. 62.

[62]　　　　　Although s. 44 of the WHSCA has the effect of regulating a maritime negligence law issue, it neither alters the uniformity of Canadian maritime law nor restricts Parliament's ability to determine who may possess a cause of action under the MLA. Despite their inability to initiate the maritime negligence action provided for by s. 6(2) of the MLA, parties in the position of the Ryan Estates still receive compensation for the accident in question (albeit through a different mechanism and from a different source).

[63]　　　　　That s. 44 of the WHSCA does not impair the federal power over navigation and shipping is further illustrated by the fact that workers' compensation schemes have been applied to the maritime context for nearly a century, starting with the Privy Council's 1919 decision in Canadian Pacific Railway. See also Sincennes-McNaughton Lines, Ltd. v. Bruneau, 1924 CanLII 66 (SCC), [1924] S.C.R. 168; Bonavista Cold Storage Co. v. Walters (1959), 20 D.L.R. (2d) 744 (Ex. Ct.); Paré v. Rail & Water Terminal (Quebec) Inc., [1978] 1 F.C. 23 (T.D.); and Laboucane v. Brooks, 2003 BCSC 1247 (CanLII), 2003 BCSC 1247, 17 B.C.L.R. (4th) 20.

[64]　　　　　We acknowledge that this Court in Ordon held that interjurisdictional immunity applies where a provincial statute of general application has the effect of indirectly regulating a maritime negligence law issue. However, Ordon predates Canadian Western Bank and COPA, which clarified the two-step test for interjurisdictional immunity and set the necessary level of intrusion into the relevant core at "impairs" instead of "affects". Accordingly, Ordon does not apply the two-step test for interjurisdictional immunity developed in Western Bank and COPA nor the notion of impairment of the federal core which is now necessary to trigger the application of interjurisdictional immunity: see Ordon, at para. 81. Although s. 44 of the WHSCA may affect the exercise of the federal power over navigation and shipping, this level of intrusion into the federal power is insufficient to trigger interjurisdictional immunity. The intrusion of s. 44 is not significant or serious when one considers the breadth of the federal power over navigation and shipping, the absence of an impact on the uniformity of Canadian maritime law, and the historical application of workers' compensation

schemes in the maritime context. For these reasons, s. 44 of the WHSCA does not impair the federal power over navigation and shipping. Interjurisdictional immunity does not apply here. We must now consider the doctrine of federal paramountcy that the Ryan Estates also invoke.

(2)   Federal Paramountcy

[65]   According to the doctrine of federal paramountcy, "when the operational effects of provincial legislation are incompatible with federal legislation, the federal legislation must prevail and the provincial legislation is rendered inoperative to the extent of the incompatibility": Canadian Western Bank, at para. 69. Federal paramountcy applies "not only to cases in which the provincial legislature has legislated pursuant to its ancillary power to trench on an area of federal jurisdiction, but also to situations in which the provincial legislature acts within its primary powers, and Parliament pursuant to its ancillary powers": Canadian Western Bank, at para. 69.

[66]   Federal paramountcy applies where there is an inconsistency between a valid federal legislative enactment and a valid provincial legislative enactment. The doctrine does not apply to an inconsistency between the common law and a valid legislative enactment. This is unlike interjurisdictional immunity, which protects the core of the "exclusive classes of subject" created by ss. 91 and 92 of the Constitution Act, 1867 even if the relevant legislative authority has yet to be exercised: Canadian Western Bank, at para. 34. The Chief Justice contrasted the two doctrines in COPA:

Unlike interjurisdictional immunity, which is concerned with the scope of the federal power, paramountcy deals with the way in which that power is exercised. Paramountcy is relevant where there is conflicting federal and provincial legislation. [para. 62; emphasis in original.]

[67]   In Bisaillon v. Keable, 1983 CanLII 26 (SCC), [1983] 2 S.C.R. 60, Beetz J. considered that federal paramountcy may apply to an inconsistency between a valid provincial legislative enactment and a rule of the common law in a field of federal jurisdiction. But, we are aware of no case in which the doctrine was applied to common law. Bisaillon itself was a case which essentially raised issues of interjurisdictional immunity. Moreover, Bisaillon does not include a reference to the leading case on federal paramountcy at the time: Multiple Access Ltd. v. McCutcheon, 1982 CanLII 55 (SCC), [1982] 2 S.C.R. 161, where Dickson J. stated that "the doctrine of paramountcy applies where there is a federal law and a provincial law which are (1) each valid and (2) inconsistent" (p. 168). This Court's subsequent jurisprudence has affirmed this formulation of the test for federal paramountcy: Bank of Montreal v. Hall, 1990 CanLII 157 (SCC), [1990] 1 S.C.R. 121, at p. 151; R. v. Felawka, 1993 CanLII 36 (SCC), [1993] 4 S.C.R. 199, at p. 215-16; Rothmans, Benson & Hedges Inc. v. Saskatchewan, 2005 SCC 13 (CanLII), 2005 SCC 13, [2005] 1 S.C.R. 188, at para. 11; Canadian Western Bank, at para. 69; Lafarge Canada Inc., at para. 76; COPA, at para. 62.

[68]		The validity of the two legislative enactments relevant in this appeal is not disputed. At issue is whether they are inconsistent. Inconsistency can arise from two different forms of conflict between the federal and provincial legislation: COPA, at para. 64. The first is described by Dickson J. in Multiple Access Ltd., at p. 191, where he stated:

In principle, there would seem to be no good reasons to speak of paramountcy and preclusion except where there is actual conflict in operation as where one enactment says "yes" and the other says "no"; "the same citizens are being told to do inconsistent things"; compliance with one is defiance of the other.

Where the federal statute says "yes" and the provincial statute says "no", or vice versa, compliance with one statute means a violation of the other statute. It is the archetypical operational conflict.

[69]		The second form of conflict is when the provincial law frustrates the purpose of the federal law: Bank of Montreal; Law Society of British Columbia v. Mangat, 2001 SCC 67 (CanLII), 2001 SCC 67, [2001] 3 S.C.R. 113; Rothmans, Benson & Hedges Inc.; Canadian Western Bank, at para. 73. The "fact that Parliament has legislated in respect of a matter does not lead to the presumption that in so doing it intended to rule out any possible provincial action in respect of that subject": Canadian Western Bank, at para. 74. Courts must not forget the fundamental rule of constitutional interpretation: "[w]hen a federal statute can be properly interpreted so as not to interfere with a provincial statute, such an interpretation is to be applied in preference to another applicable construction which would bring about a conflict between the two statutes": Canadian Western Bank, at para. 75, citing Attorney General of Canada v. Law Society of British Columbia, 1982 CanLII 29 (SCC), [1982] 2 S.C.R. 307, at p. 356. The "standard for invalidating provincial legislation on the basis of frustration of federal purpose is high; permissive federal legislation, without more, will not establish that a federal purpose is frustrated when provincial legislation restricts the scope of the federal permission": COPA, at para. 66.

[70]		We are of the view that federal paramountcy does not apply in this case, under a proper interpretation of the MLA.

[71]		The appellants argue (and the dissenting Court of Appeal judge agreed) that no conflict arises between the provincial and federal statutes because the latter does not grant a right of action to the Ryan Estates in the circumstances of this case. Under s. 6(2) of the MLA, dependants "may" start an action only if the person died "under circumstances that would have entitled the person, if not deceased, to recover damages".

[72]		On its face, s. 6(2) of the MLA deals with tort. It concerns a claim of negligence under Canadian maritime law. When read in the context of the preceding

sections of the MLA, it becomes clear that the enactment of s. 6(2) was directed at filling a gap in the maritime tort regime identified by this Court in Ordon.

[73]   Damages in fatal accident claims were historically restricted to pecuniary loss: Fatal Accidents Act, 1846 (U.K.), 9 & 10 Vict., c. 93; and Ordon, at paras. 51-57 and 98. In Ordon, this Court extended the common law to allow maritime fatal accident claims brought by dependants to include damages for loss of guidance, care and companionship, and to allow claims to be brought by dependants of persons injured but not killed in maritime accidents: paras. 98-103. None of these claims were available under the Canada Shipping Act. Parliament codified these reforms in s. 6 of the MLA. Section 4 of the MLA went further and expanded the class of eligible dependants in maritime accident claims to include siblings, a reform which this Court refused to make: see Ordon, at para. 106.

[74]   Section 5 of the MLA states that Part 1 of the statute, in which s. 6(2) is located,

applies in respect of a claim that is made or a remedy that is sought under or by virtue of Canadian maritime law, as defined in the Federal Courts Act, or any other law of Canada in relation to any matter coming within the class of navigation and shipping.

[75]   Read together with s. 5 of the MLA, it is clear that s. 6(2) provides a cause of action to the dependants of a person who dies by the fault or negligence of others in a maritime context that is to be adjudicated under Canadian maritime law. However, we conclude that s. 6(2) of the MLA, read in light of the broader statutory context, makes room for the operation of provincial workers' compensation schemes.

[76]   In our view, the WHSCA and the MLA can operate side by side without conflict. Indeed, s. 6(2) of the MLA provides that a dependant may bring a claim "under circumstances that would have entitled the person, if not deceased, to recover damages". We agree with Welsh J.A. at the Court of Appeal that this language suggests that there are situations where a dependant is not allowed to bring an action pursuant to s. 6(2) of the MLA. Such a situation occurs where a statutory provision — such as s. 44 of the WHSCA — prohibits litigation because compensation has already been awarded under a workers' compensation scheme.

[77]   Under the modern approach to statutory interpretation, "the words of an Act are to be read in their entire context and in their grammatical and ordinary sense harmoniously with the scheme of the Act, the object of the Act, and the intention of Parliament": E. A. Driedger, Construction of Statutes (2nd ed. 1983), at p. 87; Bell ExpressVu Limited Partnership v. Rex, 2002 SCC 42 (CanLII), 2002 SCC 42, [2002] 2 S.C.R. 559, at para. 26. Taking this approach, the text of s. 6(2) accommodates the statutory bar in s. 44 of the WHSCA. The Ryan brothers' death occurred "under circumstances" that would have disentitled them from recovering damages "if not deceased" because, had they lived, s. 44 of the WHSCA would have applied. The Ryan

Estates received compensation — and therefore became subject to the statutory bar in s. 44 — because the Ryan brothers succumbed to an injury for which they would have received compensation had they lived: s. 43(1) of the WHSCA. If the Ryan brothers had received compensation, the statutory bar in s. 44 would have applied to them for the same reasons that the Commission concluded it applied to the Ryan Estates. The application of s. 44 to the Ryan brothers, had they lived, means that their dependants have no recourse to s. 6(2) of the MLA. On this reading, there is no conflict between the two statutes.

[78]   Had the Ryan brothers survived, neither interjurisdictional immunity nor federal paramountcy would apply so as to render the statutory bar in s. 44 of the WHSCA constitutionally inapplicable or inoperative. Interjurisdictional immunity would not apply for the same reasons that it does not apply to the circumstances of this appeal. As discussed earlier, federal paramountcy only applies where there is an inconsistency between two valid legislative enactments — one federal and one provincial. It does not apply to an inconsistency between the common law and a valid provincial legislative enactment. Accordingly, if the Ryan brothers had survived and sought damages in tort, federal paramountcy would not have applied to render the statutory bar in s. 44 inoperative.

[79]   An interpretation recognizing the absence of conflict between the statutes is borne out by the broader context, the scheme and object of the MLA and Parliament's intent. Although it is evident that Parliament enacted the MLA to expand the maritime tort regime, two additional factors demonstrate that the MLA and workers' compensation schemes — federal and provincial — are meant to operate harmoniously.

[80]   First, an interpretation of s. 6(2) of the MLA that makes room for s. 44 of the WHSCA ensures consistency with the two federal workers' compensation schemes described earlier: the GECA and the MSCA. The dependants of a deceased employee covered by the GECA could not sue Her Majesty under s. 6(2) of the MLA if the employee's death occurred in a maritime context. Indeed, s. 12 of the GECA bars any claim against Her Majesty. Likewise, the dependants of a deceased employee that falls under the MSCA and are therefore entitled to compensation under that Act could not bring a claim under s. 6(2) of the MLA due to the statutory bar in s. 13 of the MSCA.

[81]   There is a presumption that Parliament does not enact related statutes that are inconsistent with one another: Reference re Broadcasting Regulatory Policy CRTC 2010-167 and Broadcasting Order CRTC 2010-168, 2012 SCC 68 (CanLII), 2012 SCC 68, [2012] 3 S.C.R. 489, at paras. 38 and 61; 65302 British Columbia Ltd. v. Canada, 1999 CanLII 639 (SCC), [1999] 3 S.C.R. 804, at para. 7. It would be inconsistent for Parliament to enact statutory bars in the GECA and the MSCA that do not preclude a negligence action under s. 6(2) of the MLA. These provisions must be interpreted harmoniously. Section 6(2) of the MLA, which allows dependants of a deceased person to sue if the death occurred "under circumstances that would have entitled" the deceased to recover damages if he or she had lived, can exist alongside the GECA and the MSCA without inconsistency if interpreted to mean that the application of

a statutory bar in a workers' compensation scheme is a circumstance that disentitles the deceased person from being able to recover damages. If this Court were to conclude that s. 6(2) of the MLA did not accommodate the statutory bar in s. 44 of the WHSCA, it would necessarily be saying that s. 6(2) of the MLA also does not accommodate the statutory bars in the GECA and the MSCA. Based on the presumption of consistency, this cannot be.

[82]   Second, the WHSCA and the MLA are distinct in purpose and nature: the first provides no-fault insurance benefits for workplace-related injury and the second is a statutory tort regime. In Workers' Compensation Appeal Board v. Penney (1980), 38 N.S.R. (2d) 623 (C.A.), Jones J.A. stated that "the principles of tort law have no application to workmen's compensation legislation" (para. 13). In Ferneyhough v. Workers' Compensation Appeals Tribunal, 2000 NSCA 121 (CanLII), 2000 NSCA 121, 189 N.S.R. (2d) 76, Cromwell J.A. (as he then was) considered that statement:

Of course, one of the purposes of a workers' compensation scheme is to take compensation for work injury and occupational disease out of the fault based tort system. Concepts such as "fault" and "damages", so central to tort law, are not consistent with the purposes of the workers' compensation scheme. It was in this general sense that Jones, J.A., stated that tort law principles do not apply to the workers' compensation system. [para. 15]

More recently, Cromwell J.A. stated that "[t]he overall purpose of workers' compensation legislation is to take decisions about compensation for workplace injuries out of the tort system and out of the courts": Nova Scotia (Minister of Transportation and Public Works) v. Workers' Compensation Appeals Tribunal, 2005 NSCA 62 (CanLII), 2005 NSCA 62, 231 N.S.R. (2d) 390, at para. 20.

[83]   The WHSCA removes compensation for workplace injury from the tort system, of which the MLA is a part. This is accomplished by the statutory bar in s. 44, which takes away a worker's right to sue in tort. The WHSCA is "a comprehensive scheme for resolving workers' compensation disputes" in Newfoundland and Labrador, "notably by barring access to the courts in cases covered by the Act": Nova Scotia (Workers' Compensation Board) v. Martin, 2003 SCC 54 (CanLII), 2003 SCC 54, [2003] 2 S.C.R. 504, at para. 52. As such, for the purposes of s. 6(2) of the MLA, a deceased worker whose dependants are entitled to compensation under the WHSCA is a person who died "under circumstances" that would not have entitled the worker to recover damages if he or she had lived.

[84]   As to whether federal paramountcy applies on the basis of the WHSCA frustrating a federal purpose, s. 6(2) of the MLA was enacted to expand the range of claimants who could start an action in maritime negligence law. The WHSCA, which establishes a no-fault regime to compensate for workplace-related injury, does not frustrate that purpose. It simply provides for a different regime for compensation that is distinct and separate from tort. Moreover, the language in s. 6(2) of the MLA is

permissive; a dependant "may" bring an action. The high standard for applying paramountcy on the basis of the frustration of a federal purpose is not met here. Indeed, applying the statutory bar and ensuring a consistent application of the workers' compensation schemes at the federal and provincial levels appears to reflect the longstanding intention of Parliament through the development of these schemes.

V. Conclusion

[85]   Section 44 of the WHSCA applies on the facts of this case. Interjurisdictional immunity and federal paramountcy do not apply in this case. Section 44 of the WHSCA is therefore applicable and operative. The appeal is allowed. The Ryan Estates' claims are barred by s. 44 of the WHSCA and their action is dismissed. There will be no order as to costs.

[86]   The constitutional questions are answered as follows:

1. Is s. 44 of the Workplace Health, Safety and Compensation Act, R.S.N.L. 1990, c. W-11, constitutionally inoperative in respect of federal maritime negligence claims made pursuant to s. 6 of the Marine Liability Act, S.C. 2001, c. 6, by reason of the doctrine of federal paramountcy?

No.

2. Is s. 44 of the Workplace Health, Safety and Compensation Act, R.S.N.L. 1990, c. W-11, constitutionally inapplicable to federal maritime negligence claims made pursuant to s. 6 of the Marine Liability Act, S.C. 2001, c. 6, by reason of the doctrine of interjurisdictional immunity?

No.

Appeal allowed.

Other work by these authors

2003 Category: Non-Fiction
Re-introduction of gray wolves to some natural habitats to counter the effects of over-populated wild herd animals due to the elimination of their main predator
Mallenby, Patricia
ISBN: 0973281324
Canadiana: 20030165210
LC Call no.: QL737 C22 M325 2003 fol.
Dewey: 599.773 13
AMICUS No. 28839674

2003 Category: Non-Fiction
Genetics - Gregor Johann Mendel: small sampling problems?
Mallenby, Patricia & Jeremy
ISBN: 0973281359
Canadiana: 20040126161
LC Class no.: QH430
Dewey: 576.5 14
AMICUS No. 29768606

2003 Category: Non-Fiction
Have chocolate manufacturers capitalized on recent research about the health benefits of chocolate to increase their chocolate sales?
Mallenby, Jeremy
ISBN: 0973281316
Canadiana: 20040054942
LC Call no.: HD9200 A2 M34 2003 fol.
Dewey: 338.4/7664153 22
AMICUS No. 28839676

2007 Category: Non-Fiction
Essays in World History: An Undergraduate Perspective
Mallenby, Patricia & Jeremy
ISBN: 978-0-9780593-1-6
Number of pages: 425

2008 Category: Non-Fiction
So You Want To Be A Probation Officer? A Review of Some
Supreme Court and Provincial Court Cases to Help Clarify the
Nature of Probation Orders and the Work of Probation Officers
Mallenby, Patricia & Jeremy
ISBN: 9781897518779
Number of pages: 407

2008 Category: Non-Fiction
Is He Our Sister? Was She Our Father? Expert Medical &
Scientific Evidence Re-define Identity, Marriage, Family &
Children: A Chronological Review of Court Decisions &
Legislative Accommodation
Mallenby, Patricia & Jeremy
ISBN: 9781926626604
Number of pages: 186

2010 Category: Non-Fiction
Aboriginal Self Government & Other Self Determination Issues
ISBN-10: 1602646406, ISBN-13: 978-1602646407
Number of pages: 334

2010 Category: Non-Fiction
Rewarding Probationer Compliance
ISBN-10: 1453862013, ISBN-13: 978-1453862018
Number of pages: 372

www.ingramcontent.com/pod-product-compliance
Lightning Source LLC
Chambersburg PA
CBHW081101290526
45795CB00006B/1943